DON'T COUNT ME OUT

MAKING THE MOST OF LIFE WITH A SERIOUS HEAD INJURY

STEVEN R. WEIGHMAN

Blue Spruce Publishing
8442 Small Ave
Stanwood, Michigan 49346
616-972-2234
E-Mail: Weighmans@Centuryinter.net

Published by Blue Spruce Publishing, 8442 Small Ave., Stanwood, MI 49346

Publisher's Cataloging-in-Publication Data
Weighman, Steven R.
  Don't count me out/Steven R. Weighman
  Stanwood, Mich., Blue Spruce Publishing, 1998
        p.   cm.   ill.
    ISBN
  1. Biography–United States.
      98-090503
      CIP

PROJECT COORDINATION BY BOOKABILITY, INC.

01 00 99 ◆ 5 4 3 2 1

Printed in the United States of America

DEDICATION

*This book is dedicated to my father and mother.
This work could never have been completed
without their support and confidence in me.*

Contents

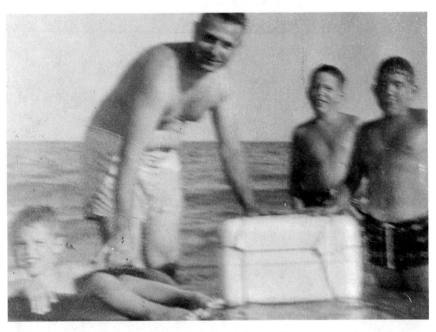

July 23, 1960, the day before my accident. Steve, at right, enjoys swimming with his father and brothers Chuck and David.

1

LEARNING TO LIVE

I was a normal seven-year old boy until 1960 when I became the a victim of an accident in which the horse I was riding bolted. A car struck the horse, throwing me onto the road, and continued on to hit my head. This accident left me with a head injury causing me to be legally blind, to have a speech impediment, and to be confined to a wheelchair with only limited use of my arms and legs.

My intent in writing this book is to show people that even if they are handicapped, they can still carry on with a productive life. When things look the darkest, if you can see the light at the end of the tunnel, everything may soon brighten up. I have heard that people who have seen this tunnel feel as though God is watching over them, and I have always thought He let me live because He had work for me to do. At times I have been as low as the bottom of the sea; at other times I have felt as if I were on top the highest mountain. This book is about a young man's triumphs and defeats. The best, I trust, is yet to come or at least those are the feelings that my heart and head tell me.

I was frustrated many times while writing this particular book. I almost quit. I tried to write it in braille and named it *The Grass is Always Greener on the Other Side of the Fence.* I tried to type, but hadn't the coordination or spelling skills. I even took piano lessons to help me type faster. It didn't work because my mind worked more quickly than my hands. Nothing helped. It was very discouraging to have so many thoughts in my mind and not be able to relate them to others on paper.

People who become disabled have many hurdles to overcome. First of all they must fight for their lives. After that they find that people do not perceive them in the same way. Society forgets that those who are impaired may be different on the outside, but they still have the same interests, hopes, wants, and needs as before. The disabled must confront the fears of acquaintances and on-lookers. It is difficult enough to face your own fears.

I found that I had many struggles ahead of me before others could accept me as I am. This story will trace those steps through revealing the problems of camps, rehabilitation centers, schools and universities that I have attended. I found that I could not always take people at face value. Some would take advantage of my handicaps to further their own ambitions. I had to learn to screen my aides and to check their credentials and references.

At the beginning, there were many barriers that prevented me from entering the places that I would have liked to go. Over the years barriers have fallen, and the public, universities and schools have become more understanding of the needs of the handicapped.

Even new technology and the computer seemed to elude me. It took many attempts and many years for me to be able to access this technology. I finally achieved this goal as evidenced by my being able to write this book.

2

BROKEN DREAMS

My father screamed louder than the siren of the ambulance, "Faster, damn it, faster!" My mother, riding in our friend Dick Wurtzel's car, cried and prayed. In the emergency room, the nurses asked my Dad questions he wasn't able to answer under the circumstances: "How old is he? What's his birthday? What year was he born? Where was he born? What's his weight? Color of his hair? Color of his eyes?"

"In a minute, damn it!" he shouted, "It isn't going to matter because he is going to be dead."

With the sound of the ambulance siren, my dreams of being a carpenter came to a screaming halt.

I was a chubby, normal, seven year-old child in July of 1960. Nicknamed Poncho, I wore a cowboy belt with two six-guns that dragged on the ground. My brother Dave and I fought to see who would be the good guy. I usually won the outlaw's spot; if I didn't, my brother would blackmail me by telling our mom about the mischievous things I had done, and that would get me the spanking stick. I played the role to the hilt and would shoot my brother thirteen times. Although I normally played the villain when playing with my brother and friends, while riding the big Tennessee Walker on that July 24, 1960, I thought of myself as the Lone Ranger on his great white stallion. My Uncle Jack held the reins and was leading the horse around a field.

For some reason, the horse became spooked and bolted. Suddenly, I was just hanging on, and the horse was going faster and faster down the road. "Hi Ho, Silver, away!" I said. They tell me the only mask I was wearing was a mask of terror. My father and uncle yelled at me to jump off, but my instincts told me to hang on. As the horse ran in front of a car, I was thrown into the path of it, and ended up lying unconscious in the middle of the road.

My dreams all exploded like a bomb. My Aunt Jacquie, a registered nurse, recognized the severity of my injuries. I was having trouble breathing because I was aspirating the contents of my stomach. She immediately began suctioning my throat, so that I wouldn't choke. She probably saved my life by working hard on me until the ambulance arrived.

The doctors determined that I had a severe head injury, causing increased pressure because of fluid building up in my skull. It was concluded after several days that brain surgery would be necessary. A decompression procedure was decided upon because my brain was pressing on the inside of my head causing further injury. In surgery an incision was made and the bone removed from my skull just in front of my ears to relieve this pressure. During the operation, which lasted approximately four hours, several blood clots were also discovered and removed. I still had not regained consciousness and would not for eight weeks. To feel useful in my recovery, my mother learned from the nurse to fill ice packs to place around my body to control my temperature. She says that she packed so much ice that Siberia was beginning to warm up.

It was ironic that I used to love winter, building snowmen twice the size of myself. Snow, only knee-deep on an adult, made me feel like a giant because it was up to my chest. But I guess when you're that small, there's not much room between your knees and chest. Now ice was now controlling my body temperature and saving my life. Unfortunately, loving winter is only a memory; the ice and snow are a real impediment to me now.

They watched over me from July to the middle of October. I was lying unconscious in the hospital bed, not needing the sides up because I was not moving. Mother was allowed to sleep at the hospital for the first ten days, but after that she was sent home. She would stay until late in the evening, and my dad would come at five o'clock in the morning. They managed to be there for me the greater part of the day and night.

My dad's cousin, Father Richard, is a Catholic priest. He came every day, as did my own Episcopal priest, Father Towler, and they always came at the same time. They both changed the hour they came and as luck would have it--and to their chagrin-- they always switched to the same hour. But, they were welcomed no matter whether they came together or alone. Their prayers were appreciated. Mom and Dad said that both Father Richard and Father Towler helped them a lot. At first my parents thought that God was punishing them for some unknown sin, but after talking to the priests and meditating, they knew that God was not vindictive, and that my accident was truly an accident. They were able to believe that God surely wouldn't punish a small child. My parents prayed, "Dear God, please don't take his mind; we'll be able to cope with anything else." This has proven true. As handicapped as I am, I still am able to think and remember clearly.

I might have been unconscious, but every time my mom and dad came into the room, I smiled. They told me to blink my eyes and I did, until they called in a doctor. I don't know whether it was because of stubbornness or fear, but I wouldn't show off for the doctors.

My parents tell me that coming out of the coma took a long time. The doctors just couldn't believe that I had blinked my eyes or smiled. It was their belief that mom and dad had imagined these things because they wanted to believe this so badly. Only Dr. Rank, who was a resident pediatrician in training, thought it might be true. One night when he was on duty, he brought an orange popsicle into the hospital room and tried to let me suck on it. I did, and it was at this time that he discovered I had a broken jaw and could open my mouth only a little. He was able to demonstrate this to other doctors, who finally believed I had become semiconscious.

To lessen the burden, my father came in to help by giving my private duty nurses a break. This was before there was an intensive care unit of any kind. My father had watched the private duty nurses suction me. One morning a nurse came into my room unexpectedly and said, "What do you think you're doing, Gene?"

My father looked up with a big grin, "I'm taking care of my son, learning to suction his tracheotomy."

"Since you insist on being a part of this team, let me show you how to do it correctly. Come over here and watch."

"I'm ready to learn," he said.

The nurse picked up the tube and instructed him in the procedure. He was a quick study and learned easily. As he left the room he turned and pointed at me lying in my bed, "You will get well," he said to me. Then he walked down the corridor and out to his car to make his first call of a new day. He walked in to see Bill Sullivan, a customer.

Bill looked at my Dad and said, "You look like the goose that laid the golden egg."

"No, but something better has happened. They have let me help with my son."

Ultimately this was one of the reasons the doctors released me. Mom and Dad were taught to take care of my trach tube, feed me, and turn me every two hours. I was still not totally conscious, but after three months in the hospital, my parents took me home. I was happy to see my two brothers and was able to smile at them. Suddenly, I was more alert and able to swallow and taste liquids, even though my mouth was still wired shut because of my broken jaw. Slowly, I started to make sounds and tried to talk. Friends and relatives came in droves bringing back many memories. The surroundings were familiar, and my condition improved immediately; I was home with my family.

The doctor who had inserted the trach came to my home to check on me and to see how I was progressing or regressing. He told my family that I would never breathe on my own.

He was wrong, of course, and surprised when he was able to remove the trach. By that time I was swallowing on my own and able to take sips through the wires on my teeth. After the wires were removed, I was able to take enough nourishment by mouth for the feeding tube in my stomach to be removed. Slowly, I was coming back.

All this time, every day, Dad would sit for a while, holding my hand, repeating over and over, "We are held together by Elmer's glue, and my strength is flowing into you."

My parents are wonderful people. The doctors wanted to put me into a state institution; they said again and again that we would never be a whole family if I went home. "Go home and thank God that you have two other sons and get back your life," they said. "Steve will never be a part of that family; it's only fair to your other sons that he not go home."

"Go to hell!" they told those doctors. "We're

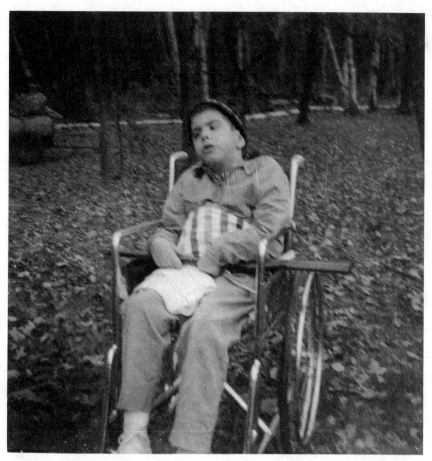

Steve just after he came out of a coma in his backyard near Saginaw. He was still using tracheatomy tube for breathing and gastroenterostomy tube for feeding.

taking our son home."

When I asked my parents about my coming home, my father recalled, "We were in a state of shock; we prayed for a miracle and it didn't happen."

But my mother interjected, "Then we realized that the miracle was that you were alive."

They both told me that the doctors said, "All your son will ever be is a vegetable. I predict that if he leaves this hospital he will not live twenty-four hours."

My father wouldn't accept that warning. He decided to look for encouragement from another specialist. He talked to my neurosurgeon, who encouraged him to try. He told him that in a few rare cases, patients did improve; he felt that at this point it was worth the gamble.

"Let me take Steve home, and he'll become something more than a vegetable," was what my father always said. I was still paralyzed, as helpless as an infant. I spent many weeks in a hospital bed, in the middle of our living room. My parents continued their twenty-four hour nursing care. Every night before my brothers went to bed, they came to join my father and mother around my bed where we all prayed for my recovery and thanked God for the courage that He had given to us at this time. It is true that we all have hidden strengths that come to the surface when we are confronted with what seems to be unsurmountable problems.

One morning shortly after I'd come home from the hospital, my best friend, Tom Greko, came to visit me. He walked over to my house with his most prized possession, a small battery-operated speed boat. Before my accident, I had watched it many times roaring around a tub of water. When he arrived, Tom was smiling although a tear was in his eyes. Mother answered the door and invited him in.

"I came over to see Steve and to give him my speed boat. He always liked it and wanted one of his own."

"He's in the living room."

Mother pointed down the hallway, toward the hospital bed that I was still using there. Tom walked into the room with his boat in his hand. He came in and sat on the bed with me. "I have something for you, Steve."

"What?" I asked excitedly.

"Here is my speed boat," Tom said.

I remembered, with some help from my family, that this indeed was a very special gift. It helped more than he knew in my recovery. I knew now that my real friends were going to be there for me.

This was not always true. Many of my friends, and even some of the family's friends, didn't call or come. We heard from others that they didn't know how to talk to a brain injured child or to my parents. Nothing could have been said that was worse than saying nothing. This taught us that not only friends and family, but people on the street need to accept the catastrophe of a family. We try to give an encouraging word to those who need it.

During those first days at home, Mother had

to puree food in a blender so she could feed it to me through my gastrostomy tube, which is a tube sutured directly into the stomach. Even though she blended a little of everything that she had prepared for the family, it still was not stimulating to my taste buds. My broken jaw remained wired for three weeks after I went home. Later, Dr. Murphy came out and removed some of the wires from my mouth and jaw, intending to come back at another time for the rest. "No!" I said, gesturing and pointing to my mouth, "I want them all out now." He finally agreed, and the remainder of the wires came out.

I wanted some real food, to smell it and taste it. It had been a long time for a boy who loved food, and now was my chance. The first thing I wanted was a peanut butter sandwich. It turned out to be a disaster; everytime I tried to move it off the roof of my mouth with my tongue, I just pushed the sticky stuff up there harder. I was so close to eating, but my mouth wouldn't cooperate. I had to be freed by my mother.

I found another use for my mouth on Halloween. I asked my parents to let me sit by the door, so I could stick my tongue out at the "Halloweeners." I now think it was more than just sticking my tongue out; I wanted to learn to talk again, and this was one way to let them know that Steve Weighman was coming.

After my health and physical condition stabilized, I needed physical therapy, and we needed a place to turn to. Saginaw General Hospital had the only program outside of the schools. My mother transported me to and from the place three days a week for an hour of therapy each day. The doctors prescribed braces for my hands and feet and special support shoes. I don't know whether or not they helped. We would get into the car and go looking for any kind of help that was being offered.

I didn't know at the time that my parents were using their savings to keep me alive. It was only afterwards that I found out how much of a financial burden I had been. Nevertheless, they say that I was worth every penny. If one really needs help these days, it won't usually bankrupt a family. This accident nearly did that to mine. Dad and Mom had their first audit from the tax bureau that next spring. They couldn't believe that my parents had spent more than they had earned in 1960, but Dad had the receipts and finally convinced the auditor by saying, "Come to my house and you will see that what I say is true."

Dad had many occupations in his youth. His home was across from a coal yard. Whenever he needed a few dollars, he would go there to unload the coal cars. He shoveled fifty-two tons of coal in a day and a half, or so he says. In the summer he delivered ice to rural homes. This was before my time; I have never seen a ton of coal or a hundred pound cube of ice. Dad went to war in 1942 and served as a field artillery soldier in the Pacific Theater including many small islands, New Guinea and the Philippine Islands. His was the only American unit to be assigned to lead the Filipino guerrillas into remote areas of battle. As a result of this action, they had the dubious distinction of being selected to invade Japan as decoy troops. The men were warned that there could be a fifty percent casualty rate and to get their affairs in order. The atomic bomb was dropped while the ship was still at sea. After Japan surrendered, his unit landed to secure the peace. They were horrified when they viewed the immense destruction the war had caused. He was discharged on December 23, 1945.

During the war my mother lived in Buffalo and studied at the Buffalo Eye and Ear Hospital to become an Orthoptic Technician. Little did she know that knowledge would later become immensely useful for her son. I am that son. Dad and mother met in 1946 and were married in 1949 against the advice of both families. Dad's work and their different religions were the issues of their parents at that time.

My parents began their family of five children, three sons, David, Charles and me. Later after my accident, the girls, Kathryn and Patricia were born.

To support this family he started as a salesman in the newly developed frozen food industry. Dad believed in this innovative approach of preserving food and became a very successful pioneer.

We all had fun learning about new product lines and the family served as his test kitchen. We were excited and enjoyed helping him, especially testing the chocolate pie lines. It's still my favorite pie.

I remember when he took us to the test kitchen at the plant. We were to test their first frozen cooked hamburg patties. Dad brought the buns and warmed the meat in the ovens. We all loved the idea of having a burger anytime we wanted one.

We were one of the first families to dine on frozen fish sticks, individual cooked pizzas, and french fries at home. Our raves encouraged Dad to approach the schools to serve them on their menus.

After twenty-seven years of successful selling, the family owned business was sold; the new owners wanted a younger sales force with smaller benefits. This proved to be too much pressure for Dad. He left in a huff and explained to a very nervous family that he had quit his job. Dad never missed a paycheck. Another institutional distributor of frozen food immediately offered him a position, and he continued his career until his vision became a problem, forcing him to retire in 1985.

In 1972, after staying home and taking care of us for twenty years, Mother thought it was time for her to rejoin the work force; all of the kids were going to need help in college. She is beholden to me for snooping around and learning of an opening at my school. I came home and told her to call right away. She was hired and worked with handicapped children in the physical therapy department of Handley School in Saginaw. She transferred to the Millet Center, where she finished out her career as a secretary for a staff that served children who were physically or mentally challenged.

3

REMINISCING

Until I was seven, I had a typical childhood. I have many happy memories of those early years. I enjoyed my friends and family.

In 1952 my Grandpa Leo sensed that David, his first grandchild, would soon have a brother and he bought us a great looking red fire engine a month before I was born. I think he knew that he was close to God when he brought it to our home: he died just days before my birth, and Grandma Irene moved in with us.

The fire engine had a place on the back for me to sit or stand. A couple of times I fell off, and Dave, who was only seventeen months older, would try to carry me home. Today I can still count on him to give me a lift whenever I call. He is the one that understands programming a computer, and will come whenever I need him.

I remember the time we moved to a larger home. Tom, the neighbor boy, came running to greet me. That was the beginning of a friendship that has lasted through thick and thin until this very day. We had many scraps and wriggled out of most of them successfully. One of these incidents took place when Tom and I played gas station and filled his father's gas tank with water. His mother watched us from the kitchen window, not believing what she saw. When it became apparent that we were really filling the tank, it was too late. Tom must have received all the punishment. His parents were too strict to ignore such a thing, but I was never reprimanded or punished.   I don't know why Mrs. Greko didn't tell my mother what had happened until long after my accident. Tom and I laughed every time his father couldn't start his car that winter. Mr. Greko never said a word to me, although I never saw him laughing.

Another special memory grew out of the time Tom and I built a go-cart. The cart was fun to build and ride until it fell apart. These episodes brought the tall skinny blond boy, Tom, and the short chubby dark-haired boy, me, closer together as friends. Tom still saw me as his best friend after my accident. He and Dave found ways to include me in their games such as baseball. They let me be on their team; I batted from my wheelchair and they found someone to run the bases for me. I never feel left out when those two are with me.

Unfortunately, there were some people who were not as supportive as my friend and brother. My first and second grade teacher was one of these. She was an older lady, at least she seemed so to a six year old. I thought she should retire then, and after my accident I really knew she should retire. She came to my home for one short visit. I still couldn't talk because my broken jaw was wired shut, and I was barely out of the coma. She returned to school and told my classmates that I was now an idiot, that I didn't know anybody or anything. How could one person poison so many minds? I don't know. I felt like the star of a freak show when those kids came to see me. I had my bed in our living room. My mother came in and propped me up with pillows so I could greet everyone. I never saw most of them after that performance. I know now that I didn't have a chance; we were all too young to understand what had happened. Many people at that time didn't understand that brain damaged was not brain dead. That's still true today, although people are becoming better educated and more aware in this matter.

I had a very large sandbox in our backyard.

One day after my accident Dave, Tom and I decided to dig a foxhole. I remember lifting the first shovel of sand for the ground breaking. Then I became their sergeant barking orders. Tom and Dave filled pails that I pulled out, using a rope pulley. When we could no longer throw the sand out, we went for a six-foot ladder. The hole became as deep as we could make it because we couldn't find a longer ladder. Then we started a tunnel over to Tom's house next door. My mother became suspicious when she saw it was becoming something more and put a stop to our digging. We were not happy, but that tunnel surely would have collapsed on us if we had continued.

After my accident, I would sit in that sandbox for hours at a time, just listening to the sounds of laughter at the school where I should have been attending classes. Whenever it rained, I was kept inside; I missed the distant sound of my friends.

One of my fond memories concerns an event when I was six years old. Bobby, a classmate, came up to me and said that there was no Santa Claus. I hit him with my fist. My parents had to tell me that there wasn't a Santa Claus before I beat up the all rest of the kids. At first I cried, but then I felt grown up because I knew the secret and Chuck didn't. I kept that secret right up until my sisters were grown.

I smiled that Christmas because I knew the

secret. Chuck woke up on Christmas morning and said that he had heard Santa in the living room. I just smiled again as we opened our presents. It was a good Christmas, after all. I loved winter and the holiday season. I loved the snow and icicles that I ate when I could find them. Little did I know that it would be my last Christmas ever to run and play.

On a different holiday in 1964, my brothers, sisters, and I had a brilliant idea for Father's Day. We made our Dad a coupon, good for one swimming pool. The coupon had no monetary value. We were shook up and surprised when he went out and bought us one.

My mother justified the expense of the pool by saying that it was for me. She told everyone that I needed it for water therapy. The real truth was that she loved the pool and it was unbearably hot that year. Our whole family spent many hours in it over the years. I can recall my father and brothers hand digging the hole for the pool. They all worked together, putting the pool up. My mother and cousins, Jane and Mary, straightened the liner to get it smooth. I filled the pool with water and squirted everyone until they made me stop. I felt as free as a bird while I swam in the water. I could swim the twenty-one foot length and did so over and over. I could make it all the way across on a single breath. I also swallowed so much water that they accused me of emptying the pool. I raced and won as long as I had my fins on. I felt as though I traveled as fast as a submarine. It was a blast. The neighbor kids came and swam with me. My friend Tom came almost every day. I stood easily in the pool and walked and ran around the inside edge. We played water hockey, and I was the goalie. We used a small beach ball made especially for that game. Our team wasn't very good, and we didn't win often, but we had fun, and that's what counted. The water took my weight and made it easy for me to maneuver in the pool. I recommend water therapy for anyone, but especially for anyone who is handicapped.

There was one thing I didn't like and that was how my family got me in and out of the pool. Every time they helped me in or out, down came my trunks. It was embarrassing.

Talk about embarrassing moments, I've had my share. While attending special education classes, part of my therapy was swimming at the Y.M.C.A. One man insisted on helping me undress even though I told him that my dad was coming. He stripped my clothes off, leaving me naked in front of everyone. I guess he never considered my feelings. I was already eleven or twelve years old. I was too humiliated ever to go back.

I remember being told how Grandpa Leo built a cabin in Au Gres about 1946. It had been his dream to own a place on the Great Lakes. I'm told that Grandpa spent all of his spare time there before his death in 1952. I learned to love the cabin as much as he had. Although I never knew my grandfather, I felt a special closeness to him while at his cottage because I seemed to gain an inner strength after my accident when we were there.

Dad always acted stunned at how much stuff Mother thought we needed for only a week's vacation. But by the time my life jacket and wheelchair were added to our luggage and food, the pile was very large. We had one of those big old Chevy wagons, and it would be crammed to the top. I remember my dad turning in his seat and telling us we were approaching Pinconning. We'd get excited, knowing we were close. Soon we were near the dirt road that led to my grandmother's cabin.

When we reached Sim's barn, where we made the final turn, my brothers and I were looking for the tree that had been struck by lightening; it signaled the turn to the cottage and the end of a long ride. Chuck and Dave always saw the tree first, but one time I felt compelled to say something, so I screamed that I saw the water. Even though I couldn't see after the accident, it became my practice to blurt out that I saw the water as we reached the long and winding driveway.

Before the accident, I remember that early in

the morning my father took my brothers and me for a walk along the beach, before either the sun or my mother had risen. The waves rolled in, so many waves and so many white caps. There was a blue sky, and the horizon looked as though the sky and water touched. Chuck, my little brother, always fell asleep, and Dad would have to carry him home. Chuck never woke up on these trips, but Dad would tell me to be quiet so that I wouldn't wake him. At that time, someone was always telling me to be quiet. After my accident, I missed taking these walks because the wheelchair wouldn't go through the sand, and I even wished my speech could have stayed loud enough for someone to have to tell me to be quiet.

Every summer we vacationed with Mary Beth, Jane, and their parents, Uncle Don and Aunt Catherine. We were so excited, that when they drove in, we all ran out to meet them. We would all start talking at once. I learned to like the days it rained; we were made to stay indoors and we played games, such things as Skunk, Yahtzee, and Monopoly mostly. Mary and Jane picked games I could play and helped me moving the game pieces. They always found a way so I wouldn't feel left out. It was at the cottage that I started to feel more normal. My brothers, sisters and cousins treated me the same as before my accident. I won and lost games as before. Some people thought that I should always win, like a little kid, but not them!

Finally, when the sun would come out the following afternoon, we were ready to go to the beach with Uncle Don. Sometimes, our cousins, my brothers and I arose very early, even before our parents, to make our mud pies. Jane and I would make beautiful small ones to sell. The only monetary unit was sea shells. When Dave and Mary wouldn't buy any, we threw the pies at them. I threw one that soared over their heads like a flying saucer. The next one came within an inch of Dave's ear. The game ended abruptly as our parents warned us that if one more left the ground, we would all leave the beach. In those days, Jane and I usually teamed up against Dave and Mary.

Most evenings, I liked to walk out into the cold water. Once, as the sun was setting, I made my way to the big rock out in the bay. I swam around wearing the big orange life jacket that my mother made us wear when we went out past knee-deep water. When we wore these jackets, we felt like big waddling ducks. I climbed on top of the rock and jumped into the icy Saginaw Bay.

After my accident, swimming at the cabin changed quite a bit; it was several hundred yards over sand to the water, and the wheelchair wouldn't roll through it. Dad mounted a chair on a boat trailer to get me down the beach and into the water for our afternoon swim. I called this rig my chariot.

My brothers were expected to help by pushing while Dad pulled. Dad had to pull the trailer through lots of mucky sand to get me to the waves. Saginaw Bay was so shallow that the big rock that we kids were used to playing on was totally uncovered. I loved to swim in the waves of the bay; I felt so free and liberated– like the sea gulls over our heads.

Uncle Guy brought some big factory conveyor belts for us to use for a path to the water. But the water kept going farther and farther out every year. At night we sat on the beach, listening to the screeching sounds of a boat whistle carried to us on a gust of wind. During the day, we collected sea shells that smelled of fish.

I never had much success fishing. My dad is the fisherman of the family. I first remember fishing at my Grandma Irene's cottage. It was a dark and cloudy May morning when I went out with my dad. "The fish only bite early in the morning," he said when he awakened me at five o'clock.

We took off in my uncle's boat, just my dad and I, until we could barely see the shore. I remember how Dad grunted and groaned with each stroke of the oars. "Do you want me to take over," I asked him.

"No, I'll do the work," he answered with more than a little sarcasm, "you just sit there and enjoy the ride."

I watched how my father threw his line into the lake. Then I followed his actions by dropping my hook with a worm that my dad put on for me. I can recall sitting in the boat for hours, not getting a bite. We would come in without catching anything, knowing what a razzing the others would be giving us.

Fishing in the bay was one thing that I missed after my accident. I could no longer sit safely in a small row boat and had to listen to the others tell their fishing tales. In the early 1980s, I remember fishing on Saginaw Bay with Uncle Jack. He rented a motor boat so that I could sit in my wheelchair and fish. A gust of cold wind came up so quickly that none of us knew what to make of it. That was when I started warming up and caught the little buggers right and left. It was my kind of fishing day. I finally was able to bring home our dinner again.

Grandma Irene finally sold the cottage. She was not well and the upkeep had become too expensive. At that time none of her children were able to buy the old log cabin. When we left the cottage for the last time, I had a tear in my eye and a lump in my throat. "There are lots of good memories there," my mom and dad said.

There sure were; it was glorious to remember the first time I said, "I see the water," when we weren't even close to the lake.

It was at the cottage that two spectacular events occurred. For the first time since my accident, I saw light and I pushed myself in my wheelchair. It was like a miracle when I opened my eyes and recognized red and yellow and outlines of people. I remember telling my parents that I could see color and form. By form, I mean I could see the general shapes of animals, people, and things. Before I could tell when somebody entered a room only by the sounds made; now I could see. I could distinguish people by size. Once, I surprised my uncle by calling him by name. When this happened, I felt like someone had given me back something that I had lost.

Up until this time, it had been hell to be pushed somewhere and left in the middle of a room and unable to move. But this day, I was able to reach down to the wheels and turn them backwards. This action moved my chair in reverse, and I pushed myself nearly thirty feet into another room. This thrilled me and now I had hope that I could start my long journey back to the freedom that I knew before my accident. When my parents returned the first time and found that I had managed to leave the room, they were happy and excited. Even though I could only go backwards, I knew that I was on the way to further recovery. It took me several months to learn to go forward. Little did I know after that weekend how far I would come.

4

STARTING MY LIFE OVER

My family supported me emotionally throughout school. About three years after my accident, the Special Education Director (Mr. Millet) at Handley, in the City of Saginaw, recommended a tutor. The tutor, Mrs. Windon, came to the house twice a week to instruct me on the cube board, abacus, and in braille. The cube board has blocks with a letter on each of the six sides. The idea was to spell out words using these blocks. The letters were done in braille, which is a series of six punched dots whose position determines which letter or word is indicated. I was able to learn the braille, but didn't have the motor skills to read with any speed. When people are handicapped, so many things can frustrate them. I didn't want to learn this way of reading, and my teacher was having quite a time with me. Mrs. Windon was resourceful, and, I might add, tricky. When she learned that I would like to play cards, she left the house and to my surprise returned several hours later with a brailled deck. Now, there's a teacher! I learned the braille and the game of Euchre.

Now the abacus was a different matter. I loved numbers and was anxious to be able to calculate. By the time I went to school I could add, subtract, multiply, and divide on this tool.

Even though I enjoyed Mrs. Windon, I still wanted to be in a school setting. I saw my brothers attending their schools, and I wanted to go to my own. After I had been tutored for a year, I began attending Handley, a special education school that also tried to help me with my mobility. I was eight years old when I began my schooling for the second time. I recall that first day. I was looking forward to that morning for a long time. I recollect my father coming into Dave's and my room; he lowered himself on his knees. He then started rubbing my head and said, "It's time to get up. He straightened to his full six feet and started to leave. I called him to help me up. "I knew you were awake." My dad pushed me out to the table so I could eat. "I feel like it's old times," he told me. I agreed.

Mother came out to help me get ready, while my father left for work. After my mother made herself presentable, she helped me into our car. We took off for one of the longest rides in my life. Although it was seven miles, I thought we would never get there.

On the first day at Handley it was difficult for my mother to leave me and was just as difficult for me to let her leave. I cried and Mrs. Lum, my occupational therapist, tried to comfort me. Mother went out to the car, broke down, and then returned to fetch me, but she closed the door and decided to let me start my life.

Mrs. Lum was more of a mother to me than a therapist that day. This special school was bewildering to me: it was nothing like my previous experiences at Liskow. I had never seen other children with cerebral palsy, muscular dystrophy, severe burns, mentally handicapped or blind students. I was overcome by all of this and wished that I could return to my former classmates and friends. The school seemed to be so restrictive. We were not allowed to talk during lunch and had to eat everything served whether we liked it or not. Sometimes the food was not to my liking.

Physical therapy, in contrast to my hospital sessions, seemed worthless. My therapist (Dr. Allen) did not take the responsibilities of his occupation seriously. I remember the day I told my mother about him. I told her how I would get down to his room and he would just sit with me. Maybe if he had given me treatments like I received later on in my recovery, I might have walked. The earlier a head injured person receives treatment, the more likely he is to regain mobility. But I missed that window of opportunity. I think that was why my mom and dad were so angry with him. My parents came in on a cold, cloudy spring day. It started to thunder inside as well as outside. My parents had come because they thought the therapist wasn't doing enough for me and other students. It was pouring rain outside, and floors were shaking inside as though there were an earthquake. It was an omen of the therapist's downfall. Therapy was scheduled five days a week. His therapy consisted of walking me twice a week, if I was lucky. The rest of the therapy time was spent in the bathroom, where he pushed me in my chair. He left and put a sign on the door, "Do Not Disturb". Other parents had begun to complain, and he was forced to leave the program.

My first days at Handley School were frustrating. My new physical therapist insisted that I use a urinal. I told her that I couldn't and argued with her about it. I decided to find a way around it by sneaking into the bathroom when she left for lunch. A physical therapy aide, Mrs. Bush, conspired with me. She whispered in my ear, "I'll help you in the lavatory, and we won't tell anyone about it." I called Mrs Bush, "Mrs. Tree" when I was young. (What a sense of humor I thought I had.) She was a second mother to me and made me laugh when I was down.

Mrs. Bush had a talent for mechanical things. Her first rule, when teaching repairs on wheelchairs, braces, and other paraphernalia was never to force metals. If you have to use pressure to put articles together, something is drastically wrong. This advice has helped me in other ways in my life. I have found that people cannot be forced either; they must be persuaded to do the right thing.

There was a seat belt incident. My therapist insisted that I wear one in my wheelchair, but I insisted that I wouldn't. I was fighting for independence even then. The argument went on for days. Finally, the belt was put on me and buckled in the back so I couldn't reach it. This made me even more angry but I decided that I would find a way to outwit them. I didn't get any sympathy from my family. They sided with the school, so without their knowledge I called the Attorney General's office to learn that there was no law requiring seatbelts at such schools. This settled the matter; I wasn't forced to wear the belt after that.

Another incident that was an embarrassing

moment for me happened during a crippled children's clinic held at the school. Dr. Walker pulled down my pants, not just in front of my therapist–that would have been embarrassing enough–but in front of other parents and students who were waiting to be seen by him.   He also squeezed my butt. Now I understand what he was up to; he hoped to discover some kind of physical reaction from me, and he almost received one. If I had known some of the colorful words I know now, I would have gotten myself expelled from school.   My being handicapped does not give another person the right to treat me as if I am a thing. I deserve to be asked before my privacy is invaded.

Going to the preschool room to tell stories to the kids was a "light" in my day at Handley. The first time I went into the preschool room, I didn't know whether the teacher would let me stay. I came in, head held high, because I knew I had some good stories to tell. Because of my stuttering, I related them on the next best thing I had in my arsenal. I put my stories on tape for everyone to listen to. For some reason my stuttering was much decreased when talking into a recorder. The stories were about a frog family, and I sounded like one while narrating them. The children sat and listened quietly. They clapped at the end and laughed throughout the telling. The teacher said that this was the first time these children had kept quiet throughout an entire story. When she tried to read to them they always lost interest half way through and scattered around the room. She was perplexed but also happy. I was invited back. It helped me to write even more stories.

Handley School was where I first met other blind students. I was taught more than braille. I learned the ways of the blind and how to communicate with visually impaired kids. I met Sharee there, and I fell in love at once because of her upbeat personality. She was little, smart, and cute. She had long black hair which I loved. She used to tease me about my wheelchair. She was always tripping over it. Sharee would say that she wanted to push me, but I had to say "Oh no!" because we always ended up running into a wall. She was always so sorry, and I'd tell her not to worry because I wouldn't break. She was the first person who talked to me about things other than my impairments. We both liked the same music, which we would listen to when she came to visit me at my house. Sharee was quite remarkable. She sensed where she was. The first time she visited us, she could get around without help, not even a cane. My family could hardly believe she had no vision at all. I liked to be treated like a normal kid, and Sharee helped me feel as though I was a typical eleven-year-old. We became great friends and still are in touch occasionally. She became a newspaper reporter, and I have become a writer.

After a year in the blind room, my parents insisted that I be taken out. They were afraid that I would learn to be blind. Their concern was if I learned the methods blind people use, I would neglect my limited sight and not be challenged to develop it. I didn't even want to use the word blind to refer to myself; if I did I was afraid that I would become blind and give up on ever seeing again. At that time we still had a lot of hope that my vision would return.

In September of 1963, I started in the room for the physically handicapped. The first year I was in Kae Schaefer's room. Mrs. Schaefer wouldn't show me any leniency and expected me to do the work laid out for me. She wasn't able to teach me to spell very well, but she did teach me concentration and prepared me to enter the senior room at Handley.

But before I entered that room, my life took another turn; I became more deeply involved in a patterning program that I had begun at Handley. It was at this time that Ruth Lum, the occupational therapist, recommended that I go the Institute for the Development of Human Potential, in Philadelphia, where I could enter a patterning program. The Institute was under the direction of Doctors Glenn Doman, Carl Delacato, and Robert

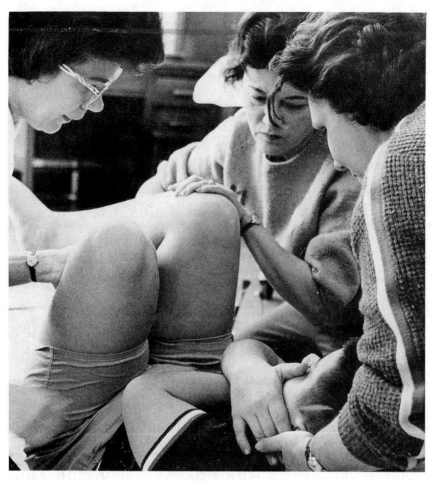

Steve put into the fetal position by vounteers at the Handley School in Saginaw Michigan. This was the first step in retraining his damaged brain in the patterning program.

J. Doman.

There weren't many other choices available for children in my condition, so we decided on the Institute. This was a controversial endeavor because the Institute was at the forefront of retraining brain injured individuals. According to a position paper (May 10, 1968) of the Institute, the goal was "to search for answers to the conditions of paralyzed, speechless and centrally involved children."

The methods were new, and approached the education and healing of the brain from new angles. The premise was that a step was missing in the development of a child, making everyday activities using large and small muscles difficult or impossible. These include walking, talking, eating, seeing, and other similar endeavors. Older, more conventional methods were deemed not to have been successful.

Even though the Institute didn't have all the answers, it was ahead of its time in search of the best treatment for each individual.

Each person was individually diagnosed over a three-day period. This procedure was quite tedious to me at the time, but it was thorough. One element of the diagnostic process that offended me was that the doctors excluded me from some of the decision making. Even though I was only eleven years old, I wanted to be in on every discussion instead of just watching television.

However, I went to Philadelphia with great hope–hope that I would walk again. Even though I never made it, I did gain strength enough to creep, crawl, and knee walk. My balance was now good enough that I could walk on my knees without

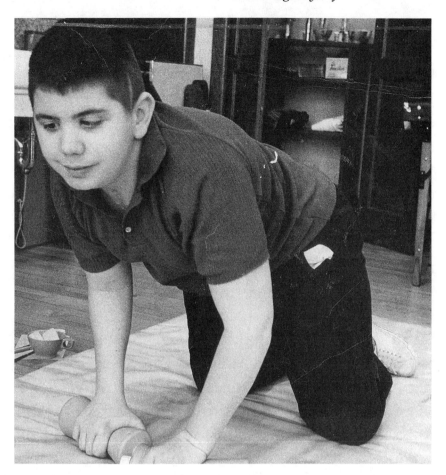

Creeping followed crawling in the patterning program.
Holding the soap bottles gave Steve balance and strength.
Those who crawl and then creep during infancy develop
better motor skills as they age.

using my hands. I do feel some loss, however,
because those were five years of my life that I can't
have back. I would have liked to have attended
school or played outside more. Looking back, I
know it was a great source toward recovery. It was
well worth it. The date was 1964.

The Institute accepted only patients with a doctor's referral and only those that they felt would benefit. One of the Institute requirements was that I had to have movement by myself in order to come for therapy. To achieve this, my father would stand out on the front lawn and holler at me to roll over. He yelled so loudly that he brought the neighborhood kids over, who would then roll with me toward him. My friend Tom would say to me "Come on, this is fun." My brother Dave started rolling toward me. "I think you'd better move," he yelled. That was the first time I was able to move myself following the accident. I have to credit my father and Dave for making it possible for me to go to Philadelphia; their encouragement gave me the impetus for that necessary minimal movement. My dad wrote to the Institute of Human Potential for a starting date. We prayed that I would be accepted. I received a date a few months later. We were all so happy when it finally came. I was lucky that my doctor would write the referral. There was much skepticism on the part of the medical community that this program could retrain a battered brain.

The Institutes received my doctor's referral and set a date for us to come. The date had to be pushed further ahead because my sister was about to be born. Mother was torn between leaving Pat, her new daughter, and going with me to

Philadelphia. My Aunt Catherine and Uncle Don came to the rescue. They moved in with my cousins, Mary Beth and Jane, to care for the babies, Kate and Pat, and also David and Chuck. Mother feels very close to Aunt Catherine; they're like sisters. Mother and Dad were able to leave with their son once they knew that the family was safe with Don and Catherine. We were finally able to depart. I sat out in the car waiting to start along the long road not just to Philadelphia but to recovery. I heard my mother coming outside on this cool February day. She was eager to go, but distressed at leaving the baby. It would be my first of many trips. We would return to the Institute every six months or so to see what kind of progress I was making. My father got us up at five-thirty in the morning. We ate a donut and some Post Toasties and were then ready to hit the road. "Let me check and see if we have everything," Mother said. Father and I sat in the car while she went through her ritual of checking all of her suitcases. She finally came to the car.

"Are you ready, now?" I asked. She turned in her seat and patted me on the head. I sat in the back seat the entire seven hundred miles which we drove in one day. When we arrived in Philadelphia and were in our motel room, Dad asked whether anyone wanted to go for a ride to see the city; this was our first visit there. I shook my head no, but he did not see me.

Mother saw me, but she said, "Yes, we would love to go." My tired dad took us to downtown Philly, even to the Liberty Bell.

Another time we stopped in Gettysburg. We drove down a long, winding road that took us to the battlefield. I saw the barracks, made of logs, that the soldiers had lived in at the time. It made me feel proud that our young soldiers were so brave. I shiver when I think about how those southern boys suffered; they must have felt so very far from home during that long, cold winter. I saw my first cannon there, also. What poor weapons they were.

Thinking of weapons reminds me of Pete Moran's tank story. Pete was one of the therapists at the Institute who tried to inspire me to walk again. "I have an old World War II tank," he said, "I'll give you a ride in it when you walk again." I was thrilled by his promise, but my father was more eager than I because of his World War II experience. Because I never walked, I never did get the ride.

When the driving became too arduous for us, especially when our trips were close together, Uncle Ted would come with the money from Aunt Margaret and himself to buy tickets so that we could fly there and back in one day. This was still a strain but not as bad as the long drive.

After each of our trips to Philadelphia, my family and others worked very hard with the patterning treatment, which was the basis for the whole program. Patterning was moving the body in ways it wouldn't move by itself. The movements sent a message to the brain creating the appropriate memory patterns that it would use later to repeat the function. At the beginning of the patterning program, I was returned to the fetal position as a baby is in the womb. When I could maintain this pose, I was ready for the next step. I was laid on a table which was waist high to the five people who would be working with me. We used the kitchen table at first; later we were able to borrow one that was padded, as those used in a doctor's office. Each of the five people took a position: one was at my head and one at each of my arms and legs. They moved me for five minutes in a crawling pattern and in rhythm, turning my head with each stroke. The homolateral pattern was the first pattern given. This consisted of moving the right arm and leg at the same time. When I could crawl on the floor in this pattern, I was able to move to the next one. This was called the cross-pattern, meaning the right arm and left leg were moved at the same time. Dad helped me up at six in the morning so I would be able to begin my day by crawling and creeping. There were five patterns, four hours apart, given to me throughout the day. We recruited relatives, neighbors, and friends.

Each day, the first pattern was given by my family. Dad, Mother, my older brother, David, and younger one, Chuck, and my sister, Kate, who at age three had to stand on a beer case to reach the table, were responsible for this one. My head was like a big rock for Kate's little hands, and it was difficult turning my large head, but she persevered and was always there. During the day, our neighbors, Mrs. Muehlenbeck, Mrs Greko, Mrs. Sanford, Mrs. Daugherty, and my mother did a pattern just before lunch. My friends, Tom and Kathy Greko, Roger Daugherty, and brothers gave the third one after school. In the evening, I could always count on my Uncle Ted and Aunt Lottie to come and help out.

The patterning program was not fun. It was a lot of work. Crawling was the first step towards many more. I had to practice for at least one and a half hours a day. In the beginning I could crawl only in reverse. After I mastered crawling on the smooth linoleum floor, the therapists had me advance to the next step which was crawling on carpeting. This was much harder; the resistance of the rug forced me to lift my hands and knees to move forward.

Progress was very slow in the beginning, but I was determined to get some mobility. I moved a few inches at a time. I had to rest often after grunting and groaning along. "Mom," I complained, "I can't move."

She would give me pressure on alternating feet so that I had resistance when I straightened the leg, "Try again," was her only answer as she crawled behind me. I did, with another grunt and groan, and was finally able to move about a foot. When Dad came home the first day I could move myself, he had a grin on his face. Mother had called him and almost everyone we knew.

"Let's see you crawl, Steve," Dad encouraged. I tried and tried. Suddenly, I couldn't move forward. I pulled and pushed; nothing happened. I felt tears in my eyes. I wanted to please my father so much. If I could have looked at him then, I would have seen a disappointed man. He had devoted so much energy and hope to this therapy and was eager to see any progress that would have made it seem worthwhile.

Suddenly, with one mighty push, I moved forward. Mother ran out to tell Dad, but he had just driven off. His spirits were raised that evening when I finally was able to prove patterning was working.

After I could crawl on the smooth floor and the carpet, I had to learn to crawl in a special box built by my dad. It had a rope laced across the top to keep me in a crawling position and was ramped with boards spaced in step-size for my feet; I push myself along using them, but there were no hand holds. This was to strengthen the muscles in my legs so that they would be able to take my weight to stand in the future. I entered the three-sided box, crawled up an incline to the other end and slid down another smooth ramp on my stomach. I would then creep around and start the procedure again. I did this for three hours a day. I listened to the Beatles on an old Victrola while I crawled. The group was just becoming popular, and I was one of the first and greatest fans. The Beatles songs that motivated me the most were *Please, Please Me, I Want to Hold Your Hand*, and *She Loves Me*. I would ask my mom to time me until I discovered the albums were about twenty minutes on each side. Then I timed myself.

Mother played an old record player when she was angry at me, and put on Frank Sinatra. I had the last laugh though; I liked him. I made sure not to let her guess that I did; I was afraid she would put on records that I hated and called "elevator music." Sinatra had some neat songs: *The Best is Yet to Come, High Hopes, All or Nothing at All* were great motivaters. This therapy was strenuous because my muscles were weak, but the music made it bearable.

My mother's earlier training at the Buffalo Eye and Ear Clinic helped in my recovery. She did my "light work," for movement of my eyes. We used a penlight or a beer sign, which lit up and had movement in both directions. I tried to follow the lights and movement with my eyes. David projected letters, shapes, and numbers on a wall, and I tried to read them. He made the slides for me in a dark room. One of Dave's teachers, Mr. Fred Case, taught him this skill so Dave would be able to do this at home.

One time I gave my mother quite a scare. One January morning I called out, "Mom, I can't see."

She came running. "Are you sure?" she asked, "Tell me what's happened?" she asked. Seeing how shaken she was made me a little ashamed. "You're teasing me," she said.

"I had my eyes closed," I whispered. I was sorry that I'd frightened her; I meant only to tease her.

The doctors in Philadelphia had long range plans for me and my family. They started everyone out at the infant level. I liked the program because everyone starting at the same level meant they didn't favor anyone. This included Joe Kennedy, the father of President John Kennedy, who had suffered a stroke; he was a patient there while I attended. I had to be able to crawl before I could creep, and they would not even let me try. I made many visits before the therapist let me move onto the next step. My progress was so slow that we couldn't see it on a day to day basis, but on I went.

My family and I hoped if I kept on trying, I would get better eventually. I made it down a mile long road, inch by inch. With every mile, there were lots of smiles. I didn't have to move the entire distance at once to bring happiness.

I remember the day that I first moved up an imaginary ladder at the Institute. I had to climb it as if it were a real one. The ladder represented the many steps of human growth from infancy to adulthood. It was charted in graph form. I felt ten feet tall when Pete Moran, a therapist, said that I could move up to the next level.

After I had crawled on my stomach for about a year, I had to learn to rock on my hands and knees as all infants do when learning to creep around. My mom or dad helped me to my hands and knees. As a baby had to overcome the rocking, so did I. One of them held me up in a creeping position by placing both hands under my belly. I had to stay up for at least two minutes before I could try creeping. When I finally went, I was gone. I went around through the kitchen and living room and back to the family room making the circle in our house the very first morning. I felt like I might even walk and run again. It was not to be though, my brain injury was just too severe to allow this to happen.

I thought that if I only tried a little harder I would be able to go out and play with the other kids, especially when they played baseball. I do remember how angry I would get at my brothers for not including me in their games. Before my accident I played third base, just like Steve Boros, a third baseman for the Detroit Tigers. So, as part of my therapy, Dad devised some strategies to incorporate my interests. Baseball was one of them which would help in my eye therapy.

I was always interested in baseball; even in my wheelchair I could still play the game. I remember the times that Dad pitched a baseball to me and I hit it. We didn't have a full nine player team, just my sister and two brothers, along with a neighbor. One would catch; one played first and one played third. I had runners, my mother and other kids. We even recruited my two-year old sister, Kate, to run when we could not find anyone else to dart to first base. We told the doctors that I could play baseball. "How can he? He can't see the ball. He must be feeling it."

"What in the hell do you mean?" Dad asked. "How could he feel it coming?"

"Well then, you must be telling him when to swing."

"I'm not telling him when to swing. All I know is that I pitch the ball and Steve hits it." That was our first real indication that I had any sight at all.

Dad was a New York Yankees fan. I became one when it was the thing to do. It was the *Father*

Knows Best and *My Three Sons* era. Boys did everything their fathers did.

I can remember playing baseball in our front yard with my father before my accident. I stood up to the plate like the mighty Casey. I swung at the first pitch and hit it into the empty lot across the street. I ran toward first base. As I rounded the bag, Dave reached over and tagged me out. To this day I don't think he tagged me out with the ball that I hit. Sometimes, Dave carried an extra ball in his pocket so he could say he had caught it and tag people out. His sense of humor was unusual at times and not always appreciated by me.

It was several more years before I had an opportunity to see a major league baseball game. In 1965, dad's employer, Bob Grant, procured six box-seat tickets for us. Finally, I was going to see my beloved New York Yankees beat the Detroit Tigers. That day came and I was up early for the game, even though it was scheduled as a night game. Dad drove the family and Aunt Margaret to Detroit. I urged him to drive faster. "Hang on, Steve," he declared, "I will have you there in no time." Soon, we were walking into the stadium. I wasn't sure what was in store for me. Our seats were directly behind the Yankee dugout at the first base side. The Tiger's public relation's man, who introduced himself as Howard, asked me if I would like to meet some of the Yankees. "I sure would," I said, happy for the opportunity. He took us into the Yankee's dressing room, but they were already on the field; he apologized for the mix-up and escorted us back to our seats. In a few minutes he returned with six Yankee players; short stop, Tony Kubek; catcher, Elston Howard; and infielder, Bobby Richardson all signed my 1965 Yankee Yearbook. Al Sanchez, Steve Blatin, Jim Bauman, all rookies, presented me with a signed baseball. Chuck and Dave were not even half as thrilled as I; they were still Tiger fans.

The rain started in the fifth inning, but we didn't leave. All of us were soaking wet and having the time of our lives. Every time a Yankee hit the ball, my mother yelled, "It's a home run!" Then someone would catch it. My mother's errors made my father laugh, and embarrassed my brothers. They wanted to leave and sit in the bleachers, but Dad nixed that idea.

In the ninth inning, the Yankees had the bases loaded, and Micky Mantle was at the plate. Mick hit a long fly deep to right field. "Hot dogs on me," I yelled, to celebrate the victory.

"Home run!" Mom shouted.

Dad brought us back to reality when he yelled, "Kaline caught it." The game was over; Dave and Chuck were cheering because their team won.

My interest in sports assisted me in my therapy. To help take the drudgery out of creeping, during the winter months we played creeping football in our living room. One Sunday afternoon, Dad went down with an injury.   I tackled him, and he hurt his knee. I didn't mean to hurt him. He tried to get up, but his knee pained him too much. He asked Mother to call a doctor. Dr. Sulfridge said that he would come to the house. "What happened?" he asked my dad.

"I was playing creeping football," he said, hanging his head in embarrassment as his cheeks turned red. As it turned out the damage was only minor; after a rest, the knee was all right again.

I was still attending Handley while following the Institute's program. Ruth Lum brushed and iced me during my therapy sessions which was as new as patterning at that time. She used this technique to complement my patterning program. She had gone to the University of Southern California for three weeks in 1963 to study brushing and icing with the originator of the method, Miss Margaret Rood. Brushing is used to stimulate the nerves of the long and short muscles of the body. A tool about the size of an electric toothbrush but with soft fluffy bristles was used on my legs, arms and fingers. I felt a tingling sensation during treatment. Icing is used for the same purpose, but approaches the nervous system from another angle. The therapist stroked my arms and legs with ice. The sensation was very cold, and I did not enjoy it at all. The way I had it figured, I had had enough icing while swimming in the Saginaw Bay in previous summers. But I put up with the brushing and icing because I thought this therapy would help me walk again.

Ruth was willing to try anything in those days. She was one of the few therapists in Saginaw with the determination to try. She gave me hope when I thought there was none. She was always there helping our family. In addition, Ruth Lum set up a patterning program for several other brain-injured students. The women from my church, St. Matthew's, along with many others volunteered to help with patterning and crawling and creeping. Other organizations donated time and materials to help. However, because I was so involved with the patterning program, I was pulled out of Handley. I spent five years on the program from 1963 to 1968. Every minute of the seven days a week and fourteen hours a day was consumed by the regime of the Institute. This time included my special meals and the preparation time for each activity. I was allowed only twenty ounces of fluid in any form to reduce any swelling that might remain in my brain. I had five patterns a day of five minutes duration each, three hours of eye work with lights, creeping and crawling for four hours, and knee walking for half an hour.

Every four months we went back to the Institute

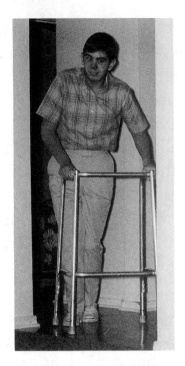

Fifteen year old Steve using a walker in October 1967.

for a re-evaluation. During the first five years I made progress every trip. I went from a helpless person to one who was able to move on his own, either on my hands and knees or in a wheelchair. My sight improved slightly. We kept returning to Philadelphia until it seemed that I had reached my peak.

During this time, I had complained of having fleeting strange feelings. I neither collapsed nor lost touch with reality. I was advised to see a neurologist who prescribed the Dilantin/Phenobarbital medication. My parents and I had no experience with these type of medications, and

I think if we had, we might have protested. We know now that the medication left me severely over medicated and lethargic. It seems to me now that if I had never seen that neurologist, Dr. Olson and his prescription, I might have made more physical progress.

One of the problems of flying to the Institute was using the restroom at the Detroit airport where we boarded our plane to Philadelphia. The toilet stalls were very hard to get into. I had to hang like a monkey from the top of the stall. This was before handicap accessible facilities. At that time the buildings weren't required to have a stall with bars and wide enough for a wheel-chair. Since the mandate, restrooms are not a problem for me anymore.

Many times as we were leaving Philadelphia, we had to take a cab. The cabbie took us down back roads at top speeds. We flew almost as fast as the plane we were traveling to - at least it seemed that way. The ride made my mother afraid of cabs and cabbies forever. I felt like I was in a race car, the action was exciting.

After completing the patterning program, I returned to Handley School for further physical therapy and the continuation of my education.

By that time I was nineteen years old and ready for Wilma Schultwitz' senior room. She was a strong teacher of geography, history, and math.

My skills in these areas improved considerably under her guidance. We discussed politics, and she encouraged me to register and vote for the first time. She was preparing me to enter high school as my friends were graduating. Mrs. Schulwitz encouraged me to become whatever I wished. I was in a room with other physically handicapped students and was the only blind pupil.

While I was attending Handley, Ron Schneider, the assistant superintendent of Special Education, told me of a camp for the physically handicapped not too far from home. As I had never been away overnight, he and I thought it would be a good to try a short separation from my family. The day was cold when my cousin, Jaye, came over and helped me write a letter of application. When the reply came saying that I was accepted, I was really excited. The night before I was to leave I had a hard time going to sleep. My father came into my room the next morning and asked whether or not I was ready.

"Am I ready for what?" I mocked.

"Camp," he said, opening my drapes, "Look it's a beautiful day; see the sun."

"I'm ready," I said.

"Your breakfast is waiting." He helped me get up.

"What is it?" I asked.

"Something you like," he joked.

"Oatmeal and brown sugar?" I guessed. We have this hot cereal almost every morning. It's an economical food; Dad revels in saving money.

If I'd only known how much I'd come to hate camp and what was waiting for me, I would never have gone. As I sat in our car waiting for my parents, it seemed that they would never come. I heard them laughing, so I knew we were finally leaving. We talked all the way there about what I would do when I arrived. I was eager for the freedom to drive my electric cart outdoors where ever I wanted. I had pictures in my mind of the rides on the pontoon boat, sitting around the camp fires with my new friends, and the big dance at the end of the session.

Unfortunately, Camp was nothing like I had pictured it. We arrived a little after noon, and my mother and dad helped me unpack. My father shook my hand, and mother kissed me goodbye. They said they would see me in two weeks. I just wanted them to leave so I could begin my freedom. I didn't know how much of my independence I would lose when I went to this camp. I started out by going down to my cabin. I was told that I couldn't go by myself. I didn't know whether the reason was that I happened to be legally blind or what the hang-up was. I had been driving my cart around for a long time when I went to camp and was quite capable of driving it. I saw other campers in wheelchairs having more freedom than I. This made me angry. I wanted to reach out and punch one of those counselors when they would not leave me alone. In the showers they came in with me and then pushed me back to my cabin with only a towel over my private parts. It was extremely embarrassing for me to travel halfway across the camp ground this was way. Instead of adjusting to my needs and requests, they rigidly followed rules that some non-handicapped person must have created. This might have made it easier for the counselors, but it did not contribute to my self-esteem.

Another part of camp life that didn't fit my needs was that the staff insisted that I try every activity. The whole day was regimented. They didn't know the meaning of freedom. There was one activity every hour that we campers were expected to attend whether we wanted to or not. Sometimes I just wanted to be myself down by the river listening to the birds singing. But instead we had to go to some activity such as pottery making.

Not everything was that depressing. They did come up with a few good ideas like a dance at the end of the week and a play we performed. We reenacted the *Sound of Music* and sang the songs. Another high point occurred one day when I was sitting off by myself; a counselor came up to me and introduced herself as Emily Ford.

"Steve Weighman," I replied.

We talked about my favorite subject at that time, which was, and still is, politics. I found out she was President Ford's niece. He was to name a vice president within the following couple of days. I asked her whether she knew whom he would pick.

She hesitated, looking down. When she didn't answer, I thought that she didn't want to say.

"You don't have to tell me if you shouldn't."

"I'm just thinking about who my uncle might name. I think it be Rockefeller." I had my answer and I was going toward the phones with this information to call WBBM, a radio station in Chicago, which was giving away seventy-eight dollars away for the big news tip of the week, and I had it. But before I could make it, I was stopped; campers were not allowed to use the phone, not even with their own money. I wasn't allowed to move anywhere without permission. They treated me like I was a toddler. I do not see why they wouldn't let me make a simple phone call, unless they we're afraid I'd call my parents and tell them just what was happening. They did allow me to call home the last day just to be sure that I was going to be picked up.

One of the fun things that I looked forward to at camp was the dance which was fast approaching. I was sure that the person I wanted to take wouldn't go with me. I wanted to ask Emily Ford, but was afraid to. And I nearly didn't. Finally, I thought, "What the heck? I'm going to ask her. If Emily says 'no' I will be no worse off." I went over to her, stuttered for a while, then said, "I'm not very good at this."

"Not too good at what?" she asked, laughing.

"I would be honored if you would accompany me to the dance."

When she accepted, I was amazed.

I was quite excited as I got ready that evening. I wore my suit and best shoes, hoping I looked presentable. I went to her cabin to pick her up. She came out wearing a formal gown and looked beautiful, like a princess. I was certain that I was the luckiest person there. We went to the dance and I felt as though I was king for the day. When we arrived, I insisted on actually dancing, standing up instead of doing my usual wheelchair one-two step routine. I'm not very good on my feet, but she was a good sport; we struggled through a whole song. What a gal! When the dance was over, she helped me back to the cabin. Emily's plans were to head to Florida in the fall to study in the medical field. I often wonder where she is now and what profession she chose.

I was persuaded into going to camp for two more years. The last year, I rebelled and spent a lot of time in my cabin alone. I was in my late teens and just wouldn't accept being bossed around. I felt then, and have for much of my life, that I wasn't one of crippled people. I was normal, at least in my head. Carol, one of the camp administrators, treated me like a five-year-old. Finally, she called my "Mommy and Daddy" to come and get me. My thinking for myself was just too much of a problem for the overpowering professionals who ran the place.

Camp wasn't for me, and neither was Handley. Although the staff at Handley really gave their best, I outgrew the place. As I was not making any more progress in therapy, my parents, encouraged by the principal, pushed to get me accepted at Arthur Hill High School. I didn't want to spend the rest of my life wandering the halls of an elementary school. However, I did do some good at Handley in 1973, my final year. I told my frog stories in Pat Arnet's elementary room. After that, I took my stories to a classroom that I was told I would never get into, but I did. That room was Mrs. Trethaway's class. Mrs. Trethaway was blind and a little suspicious of everyone. She was teaching the senior blind students, and was said to be very strict and rigid. She was kind to me, and I made a breakthrough; we became friends.

However, I still faced much opposition when I tried to leave. The physical therapist wouldn't release me. I had to see my doctor, who did. Mom and Dad wanted to open doors to the "normal" world by seeing me accepted at Arthur Hill.

5

BREAKING BARRIERS

I was revved up about attending the high school that Dave, my brother, had graduated from in 1969. And, in 1974, after expressing my desire to attend regular classes, I was finally ready. An "Individual Education Plan" was required under state law. My teachers, therapists, counselors, parents and I, attended this meeting. One of my concerns was my speech impairment. I have difficulty saying some words, sometimes making makes my speech slow and broken. I get angry at myself when words won't flow quickly. Besides my internal frustration, I have to concern myself with my listeners. People around me have to practice patience to get my message. Most people take the time to listen, but some make my life more difficult. When I am being hurried, I stutter even worse; it takes me longer to say things. People who have problems like mine experience these difficulties every day; it would be helpful if others understood speed is not the supreme human attribute.

Fortunately, the teachers and students at Arthur Hill took time to listen to me. I was the first Physical and Otherwise Health Impaired (POHI) student mainstreamed into regular classes in the Saginaw Public Schools.

I was happy to be leaving Handley, although a little sad to leave the staff that had been able to ready me for this transition. I was already eighteen years old and looked forward to being with students who were closer to my age and abilities. At the same time, I felt fearful that I wouldn't be able to be one of the crowd. Up to this point, I had resisted any attempts of people who tried to label me and to separate me from 'normal' students in order to accommodate my physical needs; I wanted to be accepted for who I was. For the first time, I felt part of the real world. My fears of not being able to do the work that was expected of other students were quashed when I made the honor roll my first semester, thanks to my teachers and hard work on my part.

Katy Ely and Todd Losee, students at Arthur

Hill, assisted me in making the adjustment into the world of high school. They helped me to be accepted. I even asked Katy to accompany me to the homecoming game and dance. She accepted my invitation, which made me happy. I had my hair styled for that occasion and bought my first corsage for her. We had a wonderful time. Katy stole my heart, of course; it seemed every time I saw her my pulse would race. I introduced her to my friend, Todd. Little did I know that they had known each other for a long time before I introduced them. I never guessed they eventually would get married. I felt like a dead man when I heard about it.

Hugh Shackelford's office was upstairs in the room where I did my studying. He was in charge of the history department. We would talk for hours about the Civil War. He suggested many books for me to read, and I read them all. I had hoped that I would be able to attend one of his classes; but by the time I was ready, he had already quit teaching blue and gray. He thought I could fit into another teacher's class, and he offered to help me get in. First, however, I had to prove myself by taking an English course, a science course, and a course to improve my writing skills.

During that first semester, Todd assisted me from class to class. Once there was a fire drill; we were on the third floor, just finishing our lunch.

Todd had to find some of his football teammates to help me down the steps. He was able to locate Dave Johnson, another friend, who came over to see whether they could help in carrying me. They all grabbed onto my chair and we started down. I can still hear Todd telling me that I should stop laughing. Soon after that experience, the school employed an aide to help me and another handicapped student. It was too bad that no one asked me what I liked. I would have told them that I preferred the students' help; they made me feel part of the student body. The aide separated me again. Whenever I did ask one of the students to help me, I was called down to my counselor's office to have the same words spoken to me: "We have hired an aide; use him." I did after that. Bill Febig and I got to know each other quite well and he included me in some of his outings where I was able to meet his friends.

Bill and I went to a couple of Democratic meetings in the old General Motors Union Hall when Carter was running for president. One elderly Democrat took his hat off his head and passed that old hat for donations to help the members of the party who were interested in running for office. I felt embarrassed the first time because I hadn't brought any money with me, but I made sure I had some the second time. I was surprised at the enthusiasm these people showed for their convictions and decided that I would be more active in politics. However, I wasn't sure how to go about it. I was still getting adjusted to the real world of high school.

I'd take a tape recorder to my classes to tape my teacher's lectures so that I'd be able to study later. I had to find instructors that would let me do this. There were a few teachers who wouldn't let me tape them. Katie helped me with my classes by reading books and other materials that I had to study that week. Other classmates took notes for me. At first Barbara Taylor came to give me my tests orally. She accomplished this by asking me the written questions; I'd answer her with the right answer, I hoped. Later in that first year, my counselor gave me a longer leash; I was able to pick my own people to assist me. They took over the testing a little bit at a time. This made both Barb Taylor and me happy.

There was an elevator, mainly used for freight, that I used to get me to the third floor cafeteria. I had lots of help at lunch time; everyone wanted to help me ride the old creaky elevator and avoid the long climb to the third floor. This elevator stopped anywhere it pleased; we all laughed a lot as we sat between floors, waiting for it to decide to go either down or up.

Today, problems with who would be my aide wouldn't happen; even later when I attended

Frankenmuth High School I was asked how I wanted my aide set up. I was grateful for how helpful everyone was, but I was lucky too that I had a family that supported me in my endeavors. My family helped me when I was down and out. There were no mental health workers, so I had to depend on my family much more than I do today.

At the time my parents had decided to build a home in Frankenmuth. Our house on Winchester was too small. It had served its purpose but now it was time to move on. I looked forward to going to school in the town where I lived. Taking me to Arthur Hill was inconvenient. Although my father made some business stops on the way, it was still time consuming for him to drive me there. Later, after the move to Frankenmuth my mother took me when she went into work in the therapy department at Handley. Finally, the school district provided drivers, but I still wanted to go to school in the town where I lived so that I could make friends there.

I had one more hurdle to jump over before entering Frankenmuth High School. In the summer of 1974 I was sent to a Motor City rehab to learn braille, to use talking books, and to increase my mobility.

Then began my six weeks of hell. My parents and I arrived around noon. Dad pushed me in; I was eager to begin my training, so I asked my parents to leave. If I had known what was in store for me, I'd have gone with them. Within a week, I was tied to the bed and the toilet.

Although twenty years old, I was forced to go to bed at seven o'clock. Since we got up at seven o'clock, that meant I would have to spend twelve hours in bed. I thought my evenings belonged to me, and I should have been able to socialize, go out if I wanted and just lead a semi-normal life. I was to buzz for the aide if I needed to go to the bathroom. However, no one came until I climbed out of bed and crawled to the desk. This angered the staff and so they tied me to the bed with a big strap around my waist. Not only that, they also began tying me to the toilet with towels and a strap. So whenever I had to go to the bathroom, I would be secured to the toilet and would have to wait until they felt like getting me. Sometimes this took as long as an hour, but even fifteen minutes was a long time. Once I was abandoned there for an entire afternoon. They never apologized. I was very frustrated.

Finally, I hid down in the basement so the aides couldn't put me to bed so early. I went down an old freight elevator. I expected to find rats down there; instead, I found the aides playing cards. I also found the reason they put everyone to bed so early. I surprised them and asked, "What are you doing down here? I thought you were supposed to be upstairs, taking care of patients."

"You're not supposed to be down here," they replied.

"Neither are you."

After this altercation, I was moved into a room with three pot-smoking young men. They smoked so much that I was sick to my stomach and felt dizzy. I couldn't stand the sweet smell any longer. I talked with the nurses on the floor, but they couldn't or wouldn't do a thing for me. It seemed that they were all in on the drug business. Dad called the administrator in charge and asked to have me moved. He didn't believe Dad when he told him about the drugs in the rooms; he said that it wasn't possible. "Move him or I will take him home," Dad threatened. The next day I was moved in with an eighty-eight year-old man. The doctor finally admitted the existence of illegal drugs and said that even putting guards on every door wouldn't keep them out.

Every day we had lessons in four things: talking books, braille, typing and mobility. With regard to talking books, we were taught how to order them and how to operate the machine. For braille, we learned both reading and writing. The writing was done on a special typewriter that had six keys, a space bar and a back space key. It allowed the blind to communicate in some kind of written form. We had to write notes to our instructors. It was with this skill that I began my first book entitled *The Grass is Always Greener on the Other Side of the Fence.* It was my first attempt at writing my autobiography. The book was shelved because of the limited number of people who could read it. Mobility classes were to help me get around the building and outside. We were given helpful hints like listening to the traffic changes to tell if a light had turned green. My mobility instructor took me outside, but not before she put a helmet on me. When I asked her why, she explained that it was to protect me from gun shot wounds. She further warned me that I would be foolish to go outside alone because of the high crime in the area. We were warned never to go out by ourselves at night. I felt as though I were in jail and seldom got outside.

One Sunday, my aunts, Margaret and Catherine, and Uncle Don came to take me to dinner at Elias Brothers. The food wasn't too good. My hamburger and french fries were cold, and we sent them back. The manager apologized for that. But it was much better than anything I'd had, and I told them that. I was out for about three hours. When I arrived back at Rehab, the staff questioned me about where I'd been. "Out," was my only answer. This attitude got me into trouble. The staff kept me confined to my room. I was also denied the so-called treats. If we were good, they fed us this crap they called brownies. I didn't get any "brownies" that day. But I didn't care what they did or said to me; I was counting the hours until I went home.

A few days later, Dad came after me. Not one person offered to help him carry out my belongings, a walker, an electric wheelchair, and the clean and dirty laundry. None of the staff was busy at the moment. They sat by the elevator and watched. When we were finally ready to go, I felt much better.

We were cruising down I-75 just outside of Detroit when I remembered my typewriter. "You forgot something," I said.

"Don't play games with me while I'm driving!" Dad snapped. "What did I forget?"

I was afraid to tell him. "My typewriter," I finally answered after taking a deep breath.

"We did forget that typewriter," he admitted. "I'll go back after it on Monday."

When we arrived home, Mom wanted to know what was wrong; she had noticed our sheepish smiles. We confessed that we'd forgotten the expensive electric typewriter. "You'll have to go after it," she ordered.

The next morning Chuck and Dad went back to Detroit for the typewriter. When they asked for it, they were told that there was no typewriter. This was a Saturday and the staff was small. "Yes, there's a typewriter," he told them, and if you don't want to help me find it, I'll find someone to help me or tear this place apart." Suddenly, the typewriter appeared out of nowhere.

I know now that no one, child nor adult, should ever be sent to a rehabilitation center without first checking it out personally. I stuck it out at that rehab center because I had goals. I had to get through blind rehabilitation if I wanted to go on in high school and ultimately college. I was glad, however, to put the Detroit experiences behind me.

We had moved to Frankenmuth in 1969. The time was right, Katy and Pat, my two sisters, were in grade school and Chuck was just starting high school. Dave had graduated from Arthur Hill that year and was attending Michigan Tech, studying to be an electrical engineer.

Leo Ott, our carpenter, built our house. He built the halls wide enough for my chair, thirty-six inch doorways and put the bathroom fixtures where I was able to reach them. I helped him by sanding the kitchen cupboard doors. He was a big man and became like one of the family, even eating his meals with us. My mother didn't like this set up. She put up with him because she knew I liked Leo. After dinner, Mr. Ott picked me up and carried me upstairs in one arm. This short but strong man could throw sheets of plywood up onto the two story roof. He was a one-man crew. I went out to the new house every chance I had.

The new house was still not completed enough for us to move into when we had to vacate the house on Winchester. My great grandmother, Hilda, maybe with some reluctance, allowed us to move into her tiny two bedroom house. Poor Grandmother, conditions were almost too much for her. She was determined to be a perfect hostess, although she counted the days until we were to leave. She never said a word of this to me. I knew how uncomfortable she had become, because she kept reminding us her sister was coming for Thanksgiving. We moved out and into the unfinished home during deer hunting season. This was the same grand woman who had moved in and taken care of my brothers for the three months I was in the hospital at the time of my accident in 1960.

It was that move to Frankenmuth that turned out to be one of the most important moves I've ever made. Until that time, handicapped students were mainstreamed in designated schools near special education facilities. The movement to allow these students into neighborhood schools was just beginning. An Individual Education Plan meeting (I.E.P.) was held as required by state law, and I entered it and asked, "When can I start?" I was eager to attend Frankenmuth High because I was finally able to meet people in the community where

I lived. Also, it was a smaller school than Arthur Hill; the smaller size allowed me to receive more one-on-one help. Once again Barbara Taylor helped ease the transition by meeting with me and other professionals at Frankenmuth. Kae Schaefer, my former teacher, and then my counselor, was a great resource and a big help. My two younger sisters were attending the same school, but we managed to ignore one another. Even though I was in a wheelchair. I made new friends. My classmates were younger than I, but I was inspired and more mature. I was determined to be a success. The professionals, who earlier said I would never make it to high school, would have been surprised. I beat their odds by graduating with honors.

I met Roger Tompkins, the football coach, and we developed a lasting friendship. He was more than a friend. With an open mind he accepted me as I was. He didn't have any prejudices. Additionally, he let me be part of the football team. He picked me up for every game and gave me a seat on the fifty-yard line. I could see both end zones throughout the entire game.

After the football games, Tom Schluckbier, a defensive end on the team and some of the other members of the squad invited me to go out to for pizza to celebrate the fact that we had won the game. Once, when we went out to a small bar in Gera, Tom and Susie Rummel helped me walk into the place. When the bartender saw me come in, he said, "Get this drunk out of here." I was the only sober one in the establishment. Thinking about it years later, I can laugh; but it made me angry at the time. I realize that we must have been quite a sight. Tom suggested that we should just go out for pizza after the bar episode.

I would have been lucky to have one good teacher, but all of them were excellent! My guidance counselor, Joy Atkins, helped me pick out my courses along with Bud Tompkins. I called them all friends. Dennis Finauer and Rick Barces became good friends and treated me as an equal. They and other "helpers" offered their time and friendship.

The staff gave me their time and then some. Mary Zehnder taught Home Economics. It was not the run of the mill Home Ec course, although it had some of those aspects. We studied about the lifestyle of the pioneers in the South. I wrote about a family who lived on a cotton plantation and explained how people made their livelihood before and after the cotton gin was invented. I remember writing about how labor intensive it was to remove the seeds by hand, making a meager living for the land owner. After the cotton gin became available, there was momentous growth in the southern cotton industry. This development caused the land owners to acquire many more slaves and allowed them to make huge profits from this labor.

Harry Weston was my government teacher, and he was a real card. He always kept his sense of humor, and he treated me as any other student. He helped me on my class project about the wealth of foreign countries. His assignments required hard work, but were lots of fun. We all had a hell of a good time though. He whetted my appetite for participation in government, even more than it was. I lived in a Republican stronghold. Little did he know that at that time, he was helping the opposition.

I was probably the only rat in Frankenmuth. I decided to run as a delegate to the Democratic County Convention. I wanted to be a part of the Democratic Party. I wanted to go all the way to the national convention. Ever since John Kennedy was president, I had been interested in politics. My lack of mobility to "run" outside had turned my interests toward politics, and I even went as far as to pretend that I was on the radio interviewing President John Kennedy on his foreign policies. By the time I was in high school, I had followed three of the conventions on television, and now I wanted to go to one. I wanted to feel the charged atmosphere and meet all of the congressmen. With this in mind, Bill Febig and I talked it over, and we decided we were going to take a bus to that year's convention, but I now know it takes a lot longer to even be invited.

However, at the time I stuck to my agenda. The first step was to talk Dad into wheeling me door to door in my neighborhood to get the necessary signatures on the petitions so that my name could be placed on the ballot. So early in the summer of 1976, I had my father ring door bells. When the people living in my community came to the door, I would explain to them what I was running for and hand them my petition. All of them signed it. I was elected, but after attending a few meetings, I realized politics would take more time and resources than I had available. Besides in the summer of 1976 I was planning to go to Frankenmuth High School. I knew to accomplish anything that I needed an education and that would open more doors for me. Without one I would be probably be stuck on the sidelines listening to news reports of the world on television, and I was desperately trying to get off the fringe of society.

One person in particular helped me. Eric Swanson, my advanced English instructor, motivated me to start writing. I had to follow the curriculum in the first semester, but he let me write freely in the second semester. To accomplish this I used a cassette in a voice activated tape recorder. When I thought my writing wasn't any good, he would encourage me to carry on, and not to quit. It was difficult to express my thoughts. I had to learn what the general society saw and felt and try to visualize this. I also had to try, and am still trying to learn to express my emotions. I am a person that tries to hide them because I've always been afraid that if I showed too much anger, people would desert me and leave me stranded and unable to help myself. This had happened and did happen many times and I feared rejection. Though internally not a passive person, I had learned to be compliant when with the public. I knew this left people fearful to interact with me, because they feared that I couldn't, or wouldn't, understand what they wanted to say. That's when I started writing a book about my experiences with other students doing the typing for me. I was getting to the point in my life when I felt the severely disabled people of this world needed a voice.

Almost everyone went to the prom except Dennis Finauer, Finey to his friends and me. Finey and I didn't have dates, so we took a six-pack out to a cabin in the woods. I pulled my first of many all-nighters on that warm June night. We talked about graduation; I told him of my concern about getting down the aisle of St. Lawrence's church for the Baccalaureate Ceremony. He volunteered to push me, relieving my mind quite a bit. He was a good friend. I asked him to go out for lunch on our last day.

We went to the Bavarian Inn. I wanted to head

back to school, but he didn't. I won that round. The good student in me wanted to return, so we did.

The following day I was at home getting ready for my exciting evening. Graduation night was one of the most emotional and special nights of my life. When my name was called to receive my diploma, my classmates and the audience gave me a standing ovation. I'm told that there were two thousand people in the audience; the ovation lasted a good thirty seconds. I was overwhelmed, close to tears; but my emotions were to be tested even more before the night was over.

The principal announced that the mayor of Frankenmuth, Elmer P. Simon, would like to make a presentation. He said that he was going to announce the first recipient of the trophy from Gunzenhausen, Germany, sister city of Frankenmuth. He said it had been decided not to bestow it annually, only when the honor was appropriate. The basis for awarding it would be "achievement with courage." He went on to say that two hundred years ago it was written that "The worth and value of a man is in his heart and will; there lies his real honor. Valor is the strength not of legs and arms, but of heart and soul."

Then Mayor Simon announced my name as the first recipient. I was honored that the city and my classmates had nominated me. I felt humbled at all

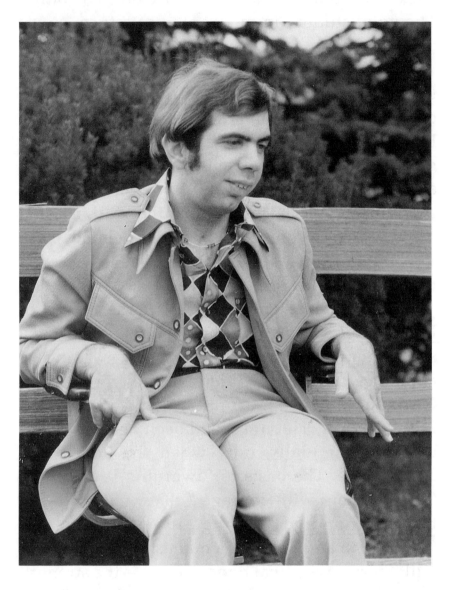

Steve's Frankenmuth High School graduation picture in 1978, the same year he was named Citizen of the Year.

this attention. My mom tells me that she and Dad cried for joy at my achievement. I know that tears were also in my eyes. The trophy is enshrined in a glass case in the city hall of Frankenmuth. The written citation hangs in a place of honor in my room yet today.

In the <u>Frankenmuth</u> <u>News</u> my mother was quoted as saying, "Five years ago we never thought he'd go to high school, let alone graduate by the next year. But we've always had faith." There were times when we'd say 'What do we do next? We're at the end of our rope,' but we've never thought of turning back. Our biggest problems are others' understanding and acceptance.... Acceptance of him as a person is our biggest goal."

While living in Frankenmuth, I had other rewarding experiences. One was acquiring my ring. I didn't want the usual run-of-the-mill class ring; I was so ecstatic and proud to be graduating from Frankenmuth High that I wanted something really different. So my parents asked our neighbor, Markita Wenning, a jewelry designer, whether she could design a class ring for me. I wanted an eagle; it was our school's mascot, and I enjoyed watching the Frankenmuth Eagles play basketball with Whitey Wilson, the coach. The ring itself is silver. It features the head of the eagle with wings encircling my finger. It meant a great deal to me because my brothers both had their class rings and because it was so uniquely mine. I wear it every day.

While living in Frankenmuth, we also had a cottage in Canadian Lakes; I liked it a lot. I took my power chair anywhere I wanted to go. Once sitting in it, I would leave our yard independently, or so I thought. I have not felt such independence since then. I went for hours by myself and relished the freedom. I had some of the best times there, until the day I got lost. I crossed a main road and couldn't find my way home. I came across a family that was leaving and asked for help. I told them that I was visually impaired and lost. They offered to call the Lakes' office to get my phone number to call my folks. As it turned out I didn't need them. Dad and David were getting worried about my escapade and looking for me. Mother had more confidence and for that reason was not worried. She thought that I couldn't get into too much trouble. When she saw that there was no holding them back, she decided to stay home and watch for me there.

They searched the streets one by one, calling my name over and over.

"I'm over here," I answered with relief when I finally heard their voices.

When we arrived home, they were all set to jump on my case. I had become very anxious while lost and showed it with the tone of my voice, "I'm tired and hungry so leave me alone." I was angry with myself for not paying attention to where I was going and vowed to do better the next time. I had learned a good lesson the hard way that day.

Another time my brother Dave and I came up to the cottage; we arrived late. We had decided to have a pizza that night. We ate it before we had the water turned on, our first mistake. He threw the cardboard into a roaring fire. The grease and corrugated cardboard nearly set the cabin on fire. Dave yelled at me to get outside quickly; the chimney was red hot, the paneling would soon start burning. He called the fire department while I began crawling toward the door. He ran out to try to prime the pump. When he came back in, I was still making my way toward the door. When he saw how little progress I had made, he reached down for me to drag me the rest of the way out the door. "I'm sure glad this wasn't an emergency," he said in a caustic tone. He ran back in after he saw me to where I would be safe. Dave was able to put the flames out before the fire trucks arrived. I'm sure our neighbors, the Ringlers, were wondering just what was going on.

John Ringler was my first friend at Canadian Lakes. He lived across the street; I would drive my wheel-chair over to talk with him. He was about my parents' age; they introduced us. John talked to me, rather than over my head. We talked for hours at a time, mostly about sports or our lives in general. Fishing on his pontoon boat was a favorite pastime. During baseball season we argued about which team was the best, my New York Yankees or his Detroit Tigers. John told me that Mickey Mantle and Roger Maris weren't worth the tobacco spit you find at first base. I would argue that they were good decent baseball players even though Micky tipped the bottle a little more than he should. He told me that the Yankees owned four of the other eight teams and that's how they got the best players, by squeezing the remaining teams out.

During football season, we again debated our favorite teams. Once again we were on two different wave lengths; John liked the Detroit Lions and I rooted for the Green Bay Packers because when my cousin, Mary Beth, was in college, she bet me a box of Ritz crackers that the Packers would lose the first Super Bowl. The Packers won that game. She kept her end of the bargain and mailed me a box of crackers from Kalamazoo. In 1997, I still had a box of Ritz crackers when they won. I really enjoyed certain key players like Bart Starr, Paul Horning and Ray Nitschke. As a boy I especially liked Bart Starr's name. Also my father had told me Ray Nitschke had a large fang, and as a nine-year old, I could imagine him biting the opponents in the rear end. John argued that the Lions had Roger Brown and Joe Schmidt, but I countered with the fact that the Lions had never won a Super Bowl, with or without those players. We both enjoyed arguing our view points, and we always went home smiling afterwards because each of us thought we had gotten the better of the other.

Other times we discussed his favorite foods or my handicaps. John liked to eat, and ate whatever he wanted. He was a man who said, "You only go around life once and we should live every day to its fullest." He never mentioned his heart trouble, diabetes or his cancer. John liked people to think that he was grumpy and hard-headed. Underneath, however, he was an empathetic individual. He understood my need for independence and encouraged me to go for it when I talked about wanting to go to college. He said that if I didn't try, in later years I would regret it.

I found out just how tough he was while he suffered the pain of cancer for several years before dying. I saw him about a month before he died. He walked very slowly and it was obvious even to me that he was in a great deal of pain, but he talked of every thing else except that.

Many times when the family spent weekends at the lake we went swimming. One weekend in July of 1979, I even swam across a great body of water. Well, maybe it wasn't that great. It was just a small lake. It was a sight to see, I'm told. Mother and Dave were both in inner tubes. I led, while they hoped no one would see them. I huffed and puffed while I swam, pulling my mother and brother. I kicked up waves in the cold water, while looking at the blue sky. As the sun started to set, I made it to the far shore. It was an exciting trip at the time. It had been one of my dreams to swim across a lake; the family finally found one I could manage.

When we left that cabin for the last time, I thought we would never see John or his wife, Effie, again. Little did I know when we drove out of the driveway how soon we would be back.

We Americans put a man on the moon in 1969, nine years after my accident, eight years after President Kennedy said those famous words: "We will land a man on the moon and bring him safely home before this decade is out." I stayed home from school on December 14, 1970, to watch the astronauts walk on the moon for the second time. Usually I rode to school with my mother on her way to work, but on that day I didn't, and she had her only accident on an icy expressway. Only the car was damaged and no one was injured, fortunately. Maybe I was lucky, or maybe I had some intuition.

I have always been interested in the space program, from the first Mercury Red Stone Rocket to the present space shuttles. David and I spent some time building and researching rockets in 1967 after seeing them on pubic television. We even managed to engineer several and to put them up in the sky. One of these rockets was a two-stage with a miniature camera aboard that took pictures when the parachute deployed. Another time we sent flies up, but they didn't survive the trip. These flights were quite an achievement, and my relatives and neighbors all gathered to see them. They were quite wondrous and we all yelled and cheered as they left the ground. Everyone chased after the rockets when they landed, and we didn't lose any of them. I still have one that I keep for a souvenir of those good times.

To this day, I have monitored and recorded every manned space shot and six moon walks. Sometimes there were several walks on one mission. The Columbia was scheduled to be launched on November 11, 1982. It would be the first operational flight and the first orbiter to carry four astronauts into space. The crew consisted of Vince Brand, commander; Robert Overmeyer, pilot; and M. Lenoir and Joseph Allen, mission specialists. Their mission was to launch two commercial satellites into orbit. Allen and Lenoir were the first team to leave the safety of an orbiter cabin to perform tasks in the payload bay. My dad wrote a letter to the space center, asking for a handicapped permit, so Dave and I could go down and watch this space shuttle launch. I was excited when it finally came; I knew that I would finally be able to visually see and hear this shot.

Dave and I took my mother's new, gray Pontiac J2000 compact station-wagon in November of 1982 and headed towards Florida. It was a car that all of us hated because it had no power. Old women in wheelchairs sometimes passed us on mountain roads.

Dave and I started from Frankenmuth early one cloudy, overcast day. Rain was coming down in torrents, and there were also dark clouds rolling in over the horizon. My traveler's checks would be a big problem that day. We made a stop in Cincinnati, where I lost them. We went into a restaurant for breakfast. Dave had oatmeal, and I ordered pancakes. While we were waiting, he asked me whether I had to go to the toilet. I did. When he helped me with my pants, my checks fell out of my pocket. We left the restaurant unaware of my having lost all my money. We got almost to Tennessee before we realized our loss and were turning back. I tried to talk to him into continuing on: "Dave, why don't we go on to Atlanta?" I had heard that traveler's checks could be renewed or replaced at airports. He looked at me with an expression that could kill and kept on retreating toward Cincinnati. We rode in silence, except for the thunder in the background and the rain rattling on the windshield. I tried to start up a conversation, but he just continued looking out the window. When we got back to the restaurant, Dave marched in and said that he had come after his brother's traveling checks. The manager said, "Yes, we found them, but we can't give them to you. You and your brother will have to go to a place where the traveler's checks are issued." We found the right place in Cincinnati, and in about an hour we were on our way once again.

As Dave came out, rain was still falling. I asked him how everything had gone. He started to say, "Keep quiet," but the sun started to come out, and we broke out laughing. It continued to rain as we traveled through Georgia on our way to Florida, stopping just inside the state line. Dave and I ate lunch at Wendy's. He ordered a salad, but I asked for a Quarter Pounder. I knew that every time I did this, he would tell me, "They don't serve a Quarter Pounder." So, I would change my order to something else, laughing the whole time.

We continued on our way for several more hours, hoping to see the sun soon. As we crossed the state line into the Sunshine State, the sky lived up to its name. We were in Florida and I said, "I think that I smell the ocean."

"Maybe we should stop and have a look," Dave said, "if you want to."

"That would be all right with me," I said

hopefully.

He took my wheelchair out of the car, and we started toward the ocean through the sand. He yanked and pulled until he was red in the face. David doesn't like to lose, but it didn't take much urging to stop when I finally said, "It's not worth it, Dave."

"Maybe you're right. It's too far and too hard to drag you in this sand."

We went into our motel room, and Dave left for Kentucky Fried Chicken to buy dinner. When he returned, he looked at the desk and saw a room service sign. "Damn, Steve," he said, we could have had room service."

"Damn, Dave," I answered, "you should have told me."

My brother and I intended to get up early the morning of the launch, and we did. We were up before the gulls. We asked the motel desk clerk for a wake-up call and were awakened at two o'clock by the most hideous ringing of a phone that I had ever heard. That was how we began one of the most exciting days of my life.

I was anticipating filling one of my long-term dreams of experiencing a shuttle launch. I wondered how much I would be able to see and how loud it would be. We left the motel in the early morning darkness to drive to Cape Canaveral, a small island off the coast of Florida. The sky was bright with stars, as if to guide the shuttle through space. It was going to be a beautiful day for a launch. After driving past several small towns, we arrived while it was still dark. Dave and I finally drove up into our handicap parking place. I told him to hurry.

"If you think that you can do this any quicker," he said sarcasticly, "you're welcome to try." Dave and I were two of the first people to arrive at the viewing site for the liftoff. We arrived early enough to get a front row seat. A small lake separated us from the rocket. Other people started to arrive, one or two at a time. Only people with a special pass were allowed to be this close; others were kept ten miles away. We talked to a professional photographer from New York and agreed to exchange pictures. There was a strong wind kicking up as the sun rose, but the winds diminished and left a nice cool breeze. It was chilly, but I wouldn't put my jacket on. I told Dave that I was fine, even though I was freezing. I didn't want to be restricted at this time in this place. I told my brother that I didn't want to wear my coat because I had told myself that I wouldn't wear one while I was down south. We cheered and clapped for the astronauts with the people around us. It was as though Mickey Mantle had hit a grand slam home run.

This was the first operational flight for the Columbia, and everyone waited eagerly. Four astronauts sat in that module and we wished them well.   Loudspeakers kept us informed of the progress of the count-down which got down to T Minus five seconds and Space Control Center said, "Good luck and God's speed." I had goose-bumps going down my spine. I was wringing my hands because of the nervousness I felt for the safety of the astronauts. The rocket went off as scheduled. It blasted off with a roar, just as the sun came up. Dave and I were very excited. To see a space shot was awesome. I sat there, watching the rocket light up the sky and thought that I surely would like to be up there with the astronauts. I felt the ground shake under my chair. It felt like an earthquake, going on for more than ten seconds. Seconds later, when the rocket came overhead, the sound was deafening. People's voices from a minute earlier were obscured by the sound of the rocket, as if a muffling blanket had covered us.

"It looks like it's falling back to earth," Dave hollered. It was the booster rocket, falling into the ocean. The rocket went over the blue ocean and out of sight. My heart was stuck in my throat. All this occurred so quickly; the experience was over in less than a minute. All of the planning for the trip was worth it, though. As the shuttle went up with the astronauts aboard, my prayers and hopes went with them.

There was only one lane of traffic as we started

home from the launch site. The traffic was so heavy that I was able to take a two-hour nap before we moved. It was a hot sunny day. Dave and I went back to our motel room for a little more sleep. We had planned to go to Epcot Center, but we overslept and instead decided to head for Michigan. We started for home the same night in that gray pile of junk. We were to Georgia before I said, "I smell the car overheating."

He asked whether or not I was sure and said, "I'd better get out and look." I was wrong, everything was okay. He had the accelerator to the floor, and we were falling farther behind traffic with each mile. "Look out your window, Steve," Dave laughed.

"Why?" I asked apprehensively.

He laughed again and explained that we were in the slow lane and trucks were passing us. After getting this information, I would infuriate him by waving the trucks past us. It made him very angry; he asked whether I would like to get out and walk. I just laughed and said, "I would if I could, and I would probably beat you home." I really like to razz David; it's so easy to aggravate him, and he usually makes me smile at his quick retorts.

Although Dave promised that we would stop for some grits, I never did get those grits. He said that I was sleeping every time he asked me. I never heard him, but who am I to doubt his word, although I know he hates grits. It was a long trip home, but we drove up a day early. My parents came out of the house with a look of concern and asked, "Why are you home so early?" We decided to come back a day early, Mom," Dave said as he made his way in the house.

Both parents started asking questions about the trip. "How did you like the launch, Steve?" my dad asked.

"It was a blast," I said and laughed at my own joke.

6

DAMN THE BARRIERS

I wanted to go to college, but first my rehabilitation counselor insisted that I attend Michigan Blind Rehab in Kalamazoo because the Commission for the Blind wouldn't help with tuition and book costs for college unless I received instruction in mobility and finances, tape recording and other related areas. The Rehab in Kalamazoo told me that before I could be accepted into either of these institutions, I had to go to a rehab called Mary Freebed in Grand Rapids so I entered in 1977. The therapists made me feel like a moron and out of place at this center. They gave me tests for the blind that weren't suitable for a physically handicapped person or the other way around. I was both. I was given laxatives which I flushed down the toilet. I didn't need them, but the staff insisted that they were standard treatment. Mary Freebed was an improvement over my last stay at the Motor City rehab center and the staff only held me hostage for two weeks.

I was taught again to dress myself, wash my own clothes, and to get in and out of a shower by myself. This didn't help me at all. When I got to college, there was no walk-in shower or washer or dryer on my floor. The coordinator for the handicapped tried to help but in all the wrong places. I should have had my own goals fine-tuned and received some real help.

The next step was to attend Michigan Rehabilitation for the Blind in Kalamazoo, also in 1977. I knew that I would be there for an extended period, which would no doubt be a traumatic time. I waved to my parents as they drove away off and left me. I had a tear in my eye and a cry in my throat. I wheeled away to the main part of the building where I could no longer hear or see the car.

What I learned there has been useful to me all through my life. I was taught to cook, which consisted mostly of going shopping for foods that I liked to eat and could warm in a microwave oven. I also did some cooking in a community kitchen. For the first time the choice of what I wanted to eat was mine. Usually, I eat what is put in front of me, whether I like it or not.

As it was at both Handley and Arthur Hill, the staff had some concerns about my abilities and safety. I had to prove myself to them before they let me try certain skills alone, such as going outdoors on my own or attending a concert by myself. I showed them that I was able to handle some of these things and to ask for help if I needed it.

Larry King, the mobility instructor, checked my vision. "Can you see this object that I'm holding up?" he asked.

"No, I can't," I answered.

"I think I have something you can see." He pulled out a picture of Lady Godiva. I still couldn't see it, but wished I could. After I had my hearing tested, I had mobility classes in the building. I was taught to become aware of clues about my location and events going on around me.

Eventually, I was taken outside, around the building, and onto the road. My first taste of freedom came when I was allowed to take the buses by myself. I was given goals to meet, such as calling a cab for myself and relating the addresses of where I was and wanted to go. Once, they sent a limousine when I had ordered a cab. That was okay.

I had a class called "Communications." It

consisted of information about the use of a tape recorder and a braille writer. I learned to balance a check book and when and how to send mail "Free Matter." I graduated from that class. I was happy to be out because the instructor called me "Honey" and didn't know me from Adam's nephew.

I was sent to the Good Will Industries to be evaluated for a week. The evaluators had me place blocks in packing boxes, screws into holes, and pound nails. They timed all these tasks, and I knew that this kind of work wasn't for me. I didn't like it at all and hadn't the fine muscle control to accomplish such tasks. I took typing classes, without any fabulous results. The Rehabilitation Center had the computers that used a screen reader with speech output, but no way for me to access them. I had decided that I wanted to work on a computer and would try until I found a way to use one.

In Kalamazoo I went out every night, sometimes to bars. It was my first taste of real independence. If I couldn't find someone to go with me, I went by myself. One night when I couldn't find anyone who wanted to go, I called a cab and left for the bar, where, believe it or not, I ordered coffee to drink as I sat by myself. I wasn't having much fun, but proved I could leave by myself and achieve some independence. The real horror began when I returned to the center and found the door locked. I banged and pounded on the door, but couldn't rouse anyone. So, there I sat in complete darkness, freezing cold till the early morning hours, when I was finally missed. The staff hollered at me because I hadn't followed procedures, whatever they were. I still don't know what I did wrong. Larry, my mobility instructor, finally showed me where the emergency buzzer was located so my mishap wouldn't occur again. But, usually, Bob and Patty, both clients at the center, and I went together. We went out so much that the staff called us the triangle.

I have to mention Gene, the Punkin Man. We called him that because he had one of the largest pumpkin farms in the United States. He liked to tell us how he grew them and to brag about the size of these pumpkins. He was the head custodian and became Patty's and my friend. He knew we liked the rock group <u>Boston</u> and surprised us with tickets to see their concert when they came to Wings Stadium in Kalamazoo. Patty and I could hardly believe our good luck. We had a wonderful time and enjoyed every minute of the concert even though, as usual, we had to sit in the last row because there was no place for a wheelchair in the front. I often had to enter places by the back door or service entrance, and once through the door, I would be placed in the rear of the establishments. I guess I just got used to being placed out of sight and sometimes out of mind.

Every night the nurse tried to put me to bed earlier than any of the other people there. It seemed as though she got some pleasure out of irritating me. One night she finally angered me by insisting over and over that it was time for me to go to bed. I was the only one who she ordered to leave the recreation room. I'm sorry to say that I swung at her. She would not leave me alone, even going so far as listening to my private conversations through the intercom system that the staff could and did use. I found out when I heard them discussing what my friend, Patty, and I talked about the night before. I felt that I had conclusive evidence that there was no privacy at all and she was out to get me in trouble. I was suspended, probably for good cause, for swinging at the nurse. Roger, my counselor, and Paul, the director, called me on the carpet for my actions. I was suspended for a week, but I called it a furlough for good behavior. Patty agreed with me, and later we all laughed about it. When I returned, Patty was no longer there; one arm of the triangle was gone and so was the intercom.

Bill, the cook, and I were friends. He sometimes made special things for me. He fixed me a peanut butter sandwich when fish, which I couldn't tolerate, was on the menu. Once he even made me a chocolate cream pie after I told him that that was my favorite dessert. We had some long talks about his days before he came to work at the Michigan Rehabilitation for the Blind School. He had been a cook in the army. I told him about how I wanted to go home, but he would encourage me to stay. His encouragement was what I needed to go on there. Fifteen years later, in 1992, when I returned to Kalamazoo, I was startled and overcome with joy to see him again. We talked about old times and all those peanut butter sandwiches that he had made for me.   I also told him that I was there for computer training.   Bill encouraged me trying because he knew of my goal to learn to use one.

I finished at Kalamazoo in 1978 and went home with more confidence in myself, but without the skills I really needed to operate a computer. I knew that I would return, and they would find a way to teach me to access the computer programs that I needed to put my thoughts on paper for others to read. I never stopped believing that there would eventually be a way and I kept knocking on every closed door until one finally opened.

Eric Swanson, my English teacher at Frankenmuth High School, had been the one who inspired me and had given me free reign in his classes. Since then, my goal has always been to write, using my imagination. I had to keep trying to find a way to fulfill my dreams of being published.

When I think about making a living in the real world, I remember one experience in the early 60's at our house on Winchester. My minister came and tried to cheer my family up by talking about how I could pack gloves in a box. When the minister came calling on that cold day and knocked on the door, Mother let him in. After he shocked us by his lack of knowledge about physically challenged people and poor recommendations, Mother got up out of her chair, red faced, and asked him to leave because she had a headache. I was angry at him for even suggesting that I should pack gloves for life; I had higher aspirations even then.

I went to a community college, Delta, in 1979 and 1980. It was a located in the tri-city area of Saginaw, Bay City and Midland, Michigan. It was a good place to start. I only wish that I had asked for more help and had been able to find better qualified aides. I know now that I didn't interview enough people, nor did I check references. I really didn't have the power to do this because others did the hiring for me most of the time. I didn't have the mental health support that is available to young people now. I did have a social worker, who wasn't much help. Delta had a part-time administrator for handicapped students. Most of the time she helped foreign students, but didn't seem to have much knowledge about physically challenged people. This was true of nearly all of the places I went. In the late sixties and through the next couple of decades, very few disabled people were out and about in public places. They were kept at home, mostly because they were unable to access public sites.

The coordinator hired my first aide, Manuel, a Columbian student. From the beginning, I had an aide who gave me trouble because he wouldn't help me with going to the bathroom after I ate in the morning. Usually, I had to go into the men's room off the college cafeteria. Manuel would leave me in the bathroom many times, and then I would have to call out for help. Someone might hear me; if I was lucky I might get help. Fortunately, an Iranian student was often near and came to my aid. I found this ironic because the country was involved in the Iranian hostage crisis and I had written a paper condemning the Ayatollah, Ruhollah Khomeini. The more I talked with him, the more I understood their religious beliefs were different and deeper than ours. I was glad for his help, but this responsibility belonged to Manuel.

My social worker's only suggestion was for me to get a new aide or go home when this trouble began, but the college hierarchy didn't want to upset the apple cart. I had to take matters into my own hands. I tried to let Manuel know the areas I needed help in. My parents came to the college at my request and talked several times with him, but to no avail. Once while Mother talked to him, he became so agitated that he jumped from his bed to mine and back again many times. He jumped with such force that he nearly hit his head on the ceiling. It was very difficult to talk with him because all of the time Manuel jumped he was shrieking and yelling at my mother, and she had a hard time remaining calm and talking over this babble. After explaining my needs and desires to Manuel and seeing how volatile he could become, my parents became concerned for my safety. They told me that it would be my decision whether I fired him, but they encouraged me to do so. I returned to school and told Manuel that we couldn't work together any longer. He asked me why, and I looked him in the eye and told him: "You did help me get to classes, but you left me in the cafeteria; you didn't get my meals when the weather was bad and I couldn't go to the cafeteria, and you didn't help me in the bathroom."

At first Manuel followed me around like a spare wheel. He would tell me not to move and park me in a corner. He showed great anger, if, for instance, I moved around in the dining room. He was either overbearing or absent. I was happy that I fired him when I did. He was quite unstable; I heard later how he had chased his girlfriend with a two-by-four when he became angry with her. My next aide wasn't much better. He was Brad Fuller, a friend of the special needs director, Jean. I can only speculate why she hired him. Brad was an alcoholic. He didn't help me get to classes either, so I had to ask the campus police to help me get from one building to another. I was beginning to know campus security better than my own aides. Several times I had to thank the Delta campus patrolmen and women for their help, especially Peggy. She was the one who helped me back to my dorm many times.

I remember one day that it was snowing so hard that I couldn't see two feet in front of me and my aide never showed up. I went into the storm by myself. Thank goodness, Peggy came to my rescue again. I saw her approaching, and, boy, was I ever relieved. Jean, my consultant, called me into her office again. This time I was told to stop bothering the campus police, although she wouldn't help me find a solution to force my aide to meet me on campus and take me back to the dorm.

Firing my second aide wasn't a hard decision, for he was lodged in the county jail for drunken driving and stealing. The college sent me home for a week until my parents called and said they were bringing me back. They let me enter, and I hired a new aide, Andy Clantor. I saw him carrying out his laundry, and he needed me as much as I needed him at the time because he was short of funds. When I returned from my week of unasked vacation, Andy wanted to jump right in with both feet. In the beginning he was the best aide I'd had. Little did I know at that time he would turn on me also. It took me a long time before I could put trust in people outside of my family. He helped me from class to class and around campus. Andy was simply great; thus, when he came to my room one night and said that he was transferring to Central Michigan and asked me to go with him. I said that I would. Bells and whistles should have been going off in my head. He was just too eager to help me. He had gotten used to the money, and I should have known better. I would never hire a friend or hire in panic again.

The various problems I had with my personal needs were the biggest difficulties that I had to overcome. I learned a lot in college, and it wasn't always so horrible. I had fun, lots of fun, in my classes. I really enjoyed talking about politics with my government professor. He would let me attend a night course so that I would have a better opportunity to understand the course material. My government teacher gave me my exams orally. I just wish that I'd had stronger support from the community to help me solve these problems. The courses at Delta were very hard at times. I think a smaller university is a better place to start; I found that the professors will usually work with you on a one-to-one basis. I was able to drop in on my

instructors nearly any time.   Fordy Kennedy was
the physical education instructor. He would help
me do stretching and weight lifting exercises. He
was a good friend. Later, Mr. Levi was my creative
writing instructor. He helped and inspired me to
start writing this book. He gave me the confidence
I needed to write, and it was his guiding hand in
that first year of college that made me feel that I
could do it. He expected the same work from me
as the rest of the class and at least as much effort.

Before I could continue with college, during
the time when most kids have summer vacation, I
was in the hospital once again for an operation. I
was reminded of the first time several years before.
My legs were spastic and so tight together that I
was very uncomfortable. My surgeon told me he
would inject a medication to relax the abductor
muscles to see if a release would be helpful. I had
had an appointment for noon, but at seven o'clock
that evening he had not arrived at the hospital.
Mother was getting very hungry, as we all were,
and went to buy a candy bar in the gift shop. There
she met my surgeon, who had completely forgotten
the appointment. He apologized and came up to
my room. The test was very painful, but it proved
a release of the muscles would help me.

This time my right knee wouldn't support me.
Although I can't walk without support, I am able
to stand, which helps others to assist me with my

daily needs. My parents and I talked it over, and I decided to have the operation to repair the torn cartilage. The procedure was successful. I was at St. Luke's Hospital recuperating. My surgeon told me that I needed to go to Saginaw Community Hospital for therapy. An ambulance took me, but not with its sirens blaring. I thought that this would be fun, even if it was to another hospital. It was a hot day in the middle of summer, and there I was, riding in an ambulance with my leg sticking out like a rifle.

I was there only about three weeks, but it seemed like forever. I was hurt and angry with my parents because they had gone on vacation, leaving me behind. I learned later that a support system had been set up for me. My aunts, Lottie and Margaret, came nearly every day, and when they couldn't come, someone else did. They brought me lunch and their famous peanut butter fudge, which we ate in the courtyard. Mom and Dad were gone only a week, but it seemed a hell of a lot longer. There was no one at the hospital I could relate to. They were all elderly or demented. Someone was yelling all night. I was frightened for myself and felt pity for them. Kate, my sister, finally came to pick me up and take me home. This was a happy turn of events because no one intimidates her. She was the only one who would dump my milk of magnesia. I told her to do it, and she did. We had a problem, though; the doctor hadn't signed my release. We waited three hours for him. We called his office, but he didn't answer. Kate said that she couldn't wait any longer, so I signed myself out and left. I'm still waiting for his call.

My knee was then strong enough to enable me to attend Central Michigan University. However, my first day was a disaster. Early in the morning, Andy, my aide, came into my room and said, "It's time to get up." I was already sitting up in bed. Andy said, "Are you all set to leave?"

He opened my drapes and helped me out of bed. The manner that he sat me in my chair should have rung an alarm that something was wrong. He pushed me into the kitchen even though I told him that I could take myself. "I'll help you," he tried to say. I knew that he wasn't himself; he was trying to be too helpful. When we finally left, I hoped his word would be good. I was a little anxious. "There's nothing to be afraid of," he assured me. "I'll take you to your first class." I found out later in the morning his assurances weren't worth a damn. That was a start of a long, long day that I'll never forget.

He took me to my first class, but the problem was that Andy neglected to come back for me. So, as I went down the hallway, I tried to remember the route that I had taken an hour earlier. I went back and forth looking for it. There were several students standing around, watching me because I had a "Blind" sign on the back of my wheelchair. After much deliberation, I chose the stairs instead of the ramp; my vision was too impaired to tell the difference. But as my front wheels rode down the first step, I knew that I had chosen the wrong route. I lost my breath, and it seemed as though my heart was going to beat itself right out of my chest. I tumbled, wheelchair and all, to the bottom. This would have been a good opportunity to use the cane training that I received in Kalamazoo. I thought about it when I was at the bottom of the stairs. What I can't understand is why the students watched me try to go down the steps. Why did all those people stand there and watch me take the stairway? I think it was because they didn't know how to talk to someone who was different from them.   I can't get angry at ignorance.   I went crashing down the stairwell. I landed at the bottom, with the heavy electric wheelchair on top of me, shouting, "I'm okay." I was so ready to say I was all right, even though I might have been dying; all that I could think was that the school was going to send me home. I was frightened while I lay on the floor, not for myself, but for my college career. I didn't want to be sent home; I was just starting. I lay on the floor, looking up at all these people, looking down at me. Then I watched them walk away. It was all I could do not to cry out, "You morons, won't someone help me?" The custodian did come over and offer his assistance by lifting the wheelchair off me and calling my aide.

Andy offered no apology for being late and leaving me on my own. He was anxious for me to go to the Health Center, but I didn't want to go. I had started college and didn't want any interruptions. Besides, I didn't feel that I was injured. Andy took me to the Health center anyway and wanted me to be examined by a neurologist.

The Health Center wouldn't call the ambulance until I told an incompetent worker that he better call one if he thought I had bleeding in my head. The Health Center wouldn't deploy one of their local ambulances for me; these were on standby for emergencies, although the ambulance service had two units. The Health Service called Saint Luke's Hospital in Saginaw, about fifty miles away, and ordered an ambulance from there. The college doctor told me that I had bleeding in my head. The supervisor for the handicapped called my mother. She was frightened, and so was I. That's no joke! I had to go to the bathroom and the doctor let me. When I came out, the doctor looked at me with sunken eyes, as though he couldn't see me. If he thought my head was bleeding, he should have kept me down. If his diagnosis was right, I should have been dead. I couldn't figure out the doctor, if he could be called a doctor. When the doctor called my mother at work, she said, in shock, "If you think it's that serious, I would be afraid to transport him." When they told her an ambulance from Saint Luke's was coming, she yelled into the phone, "Why can't one of yours be used?"

They told her that these ambulances served only the Mt. Pleasant area and were only for emergencies.

Mother thought it strange that he wanted her to come after me. If hemorrhaging wasn't an emergency, what was? Knowing that an ambulance was better equipped to handle medical situations and could make better time on the roads, she said, "I'll meet Steve at the hospital."

The E.M.S. people finally arrived, and they were the same men who had taken me for a ride just a week earlier for rehabilitation at Saginaw Community hospital. We talked and joked on the ride back. When we drove up to the hospital, my parents were waiting for me. As the orderlies took me in, I told them to double time it. The doctor took one look at me and said, "Take him home with you tonight. If he seems okay, he should be able to go back to college tomorrow." Within twenty-four hours I was on my way back to Central Michigan.

My parents took me back early the following morning; we arrived before noon. When we approached my apartment, my father let himself out of the car and walked toward it. I said, "Be careful, Dad," as he knocked on the door. Andy came out of his bedroom rubbing his eyes; then he recognized my father. He was stunned to see him. He tried to say something, opening and shutting his mouth several times, but nothing came out. Finally, an awful sound came from the little man. He said, "I wasn't expecting you for three weeks at least. I thought you would be gone for a lot longer than this because of the brace on your leg and the fall."

I had come too far to let a little fall stop me, but the first semester was very hard for me because I had to get around on such a large campus. In one incident, the snow plow came while I was gone and plowed our sidewalk leaving snow blocking the cut-out of the wheelchair ramp. When I came back, the bus driver let me off and asked me whether I needed any help. I said that I didn't because I couldn't see the snow on both sides of the ramp. Once I was alone, I realized that I couldn't maneuver myself around the plowed snow in my electric wheelchair. I kept putting it in reverse and then rocking it forward, but the more I did this the more I would become lodged in the snow. My hands, feet, and face all got slightly frost bitten. It was painful, but I wouldn't go to the medical center because I didn't want to be sent home again. I knew this was always the solution that would be presented to me. I had to wait for two hours before one of my neighbors came home so that I could ask, "Will you help me get into my apartment?"

At Central, the Special Service Coordinator would not let me ride the bus alone. Andy said that he couldn't come with me because that would make him late for his courses. I still had to get to my classes, I reminded him. I became lost trying to go alone and made the driver wait for me, which in turn made her late. I called the incompetent coordinator for the physically handicapped, and she called me into her office to tell me that I couldn't ride the bus anymore. I started to leave, but didn't want to be thought a coward. I turned and came back, and looked her squarely in the eye. "What do you think you're doing to me? First of all, your kind sends us home every chance you get. If you won't let me ride, I'll have to figure out some other way to travel around." She told me to ask the city transit. She said it was that or my aide had to be with me when I rode the school's bus. I had no one to fall back on at that time; Andy wouldn't ride the bus, and probably with good reason. To get on the bus took more than one phone call, and it usually made both of us late for classes. So, out into the frigid weather we went, he at the controls of my wheelchair as I felt yet another small part of my independence slipping away.

Another time that my aide let me down was when he left me in the apartment by myself for more than twenty-four hours. I was wearing a brace which held my leg in place so that my knee, recently operated on, would be able to heal. I was in our lavatory and fell down. I was caught behind my wheelchair, between the tub and the john, on my knees all that time, sometimes praying, other times crying. I screamed for help, but no one came, not Andy, not anyone. I kneeled before the toilet, which had a horrible smell because no one had cleaned it in several weeks. While kneeling there, I contemplated suicide as I knelt in my own urine. It's one of the loneliest feelings that anyone can experience. Andy had left early that morning and didn't return until late the following night. (I found this out much later from my neighbor, Steve Smith).

Luckily, my parents came to the rescue. They arrived out of nowhere, unexpectedly. On a whim, they had decided to go north and stopped by to see me. I was so relieved to see them. I thanked them for coming; I had been down there a long, long time. They were horrified and Dad gathered my things and took me with them. Dad gave Andy a talking to, but it had no effect on him. He was the blind one, blind to what had happened, and things did not improve.

I was at Central for eleven or twelve weeks when my aide made another of the many mistakes that my parents would not, or could not, see. They thought Andy was a great guy because at Delta he had really assisted me with my many needs. They had trouble accepting the fact that he could have changed so much. They thought that I was exaggerating. When Andy talked to them, he gave them a different account of the previous few weeks than I had told them. I had said that he wasn't helping me the way that he said he was. I kept explaining how Andy "took care" of me, like the time when, like a dummy, I sat there and nodded my head when he asked me whether I would be all right while he went to a football game. Little did I know that he was going to spend the night at his girl friend's dorm. I fell onto the floor trying to get into bed. There was no one around to hear my frantic yelling all night. I called and called for someone to please come and help me. I spent the night on the cold cement floor, moving all over to keep warm when the sun came up. Andy came home with a broad grin on his face. It wasn't long before we were yelling at each other. His smile dissipated as quickly as it had come. I wanted to fire him on the spot, but I had no one I could turn to. Clint Simon, a 65-year old social worker, thought I was lucky to find anyone. Clint just didn't understand the situation and had no inclination to investigate it. If there had been a mental health person or the CSLA (Community

Supported Living Arrangement Board) program, I would have been better served.

During that summer of misery, Andy boiled me a dozen eggs and told me to let him know when they were gone. It had become his way of fixing my meals. Then off he would go into the beautiful day. I tried to tell him that the eggs were gone; he would ask, "How could they be?" When he came back at night, I would ask him what we were having for dinner. He would say that he was tired, to make my own mush, and he would disappear. I was afraid that if I fired him my college days would be over. I survived by complementing my diet with my mush. It consisted mostly of oatmeal mush that I had concocted and could barely swallow. Sometimes I ate it three times a day, while he painted houses to earn extra money.

I was a prisoner in our apartment during the summer I remained at Central. Andy had convinced my parents that I should stay and become acquainted with the campus. I protested, but to no avail. I was paying the apartment rent, and he received chore person money, the real reason he wanted me to stay. Andy left me early in the morning and didn't return until late at night. This situation depressed me. There was a sunny, blue sky when he left and a pitch black one when he returned. "Where have you been?" I asked as I grew angrier with every passing minute. "It's been dark for five or six hours." From that day on, he closed the drapes so I wasn't able to tell what time of day it was. Andy left me all day with the drapes closed; this bastard knew that I couldn't reach the cord to open them. He also knew that I needed those drapes open because of my limited vision; I needed all the light that was available.

When Andy returned home, he was no help either. He would say that he was tired from painting houses all day, then off he would go. "Thanks a lot, pal," I said to an empty apartment.

During that summer I went over to the speech clinic to volunteer. After negotiating with the director, we agreed that I could come over for a couple of hours to help. I had hoped to be useful in some way, if only to share my experiences. In the evening of the second day, Andy and I went over. My aide went up the steps to check the door for me. All of the doors were locked. When he came back down, he was almost crying. I thought the tears were for me, but, alas, he was crying for himself. He had other plans, and they didn't include me. He wanted to farm me out, but now I was still his responsibility. I don't know whether it was because the instructor wanted me out of his hair or the doors were locked for some other reason.

There were some friendly CMU students who didn't have such hang-ups when encountering handicapped students. Carol Ilku was a student volunteer. She came twice a week for her entire senior year to help with the reading portions of my psychology course. We became friends and went to concerts on campus, which provided a good break from studies for me. George Armstrong was another of the students who became a friend. We met in the school's cafeteria. We hit it off as good friends right from the beginning. I found him to be very friendly that first day. Mr. Armstrong helped me carry my tray to the table where I was sitting in the cafeteria. He introduced himself: "My name is George. What's yours?"

With a mouthful of food and a smile on my face, I said, "I'm Steve." From that moment on, I knew that we would be good friends. We have been that ever since.

One day, I met George outside the speech clinic, on the sidewalk. He was on his way to work there. He said, "I'll see you when I finish work." I suggested that we meet out by the Mission Road. When he came back, I sensed something was amiss.

George sat down next to me, shook his head and said, "My friend, I talked until I was blue in the face, but it did no good. They said you can't volunteer because of your speech." I told him that I had guessed that before he even spoke. I knew that anger wasn't appropriate for me then; he wasn't to blame. I thanked him for his interest.

Andy told me that I should get outdoors more

and enjoy the weather. He goaded me into going alone and called me a coward when I didn't. But the first time, I became stuck with a new problem. I tried to cross a six-lane highway, thinking it was just a huge parking lot; I found out the truth only much later.

One morning that summer, he asked what I was going to do. I reminded him that he had said we would go shopping. He said we would go some other day and that he was going to paint. He had taken another step toward being fired. I went out that day on my own, wheeled around campus, then on my way home tipped over. Some passing students assisted me this time by righting the chair and helping me back into it. I was able to get back to the apartment, but I began to think that going around the campus alone was probably too dangerous. If someone had familiarized me with the roads, maybe I could have managed; but then again, maybe not.

During that summer, Andy signed both his name and mine to the checks that were being paid to him to take me from class to class. I had taken no classes that summer, so he was paid for work he hadn't done. I learned this when I applied for my class transcripts and was denied them because of a large debt that Central said I owed. As I had never seen or heard of the money, I felt as though I owed nothing. It took many letters and phone calls to clear the matter up. I finally wrote the Attorney General of Michigan, who contacted the university. They transferred the debt to Andy, and he wasn't allowed to graduate until he repaid the university.

I remember another time that Andy let me down. It was one evening when he went out with his friends from Big Rapids. He said, "Steve, I'll be going out for three hours or so." Then he was gone all night. I called Karen, one of my readers, to tell her that I had smelled a gas leak. She thought that I said I couldn't sleep. It was about two in the morning. I must have awakened her, and she wouldn't come. I was becoming frantic so I went across the hall and knocked on the door of my neighbor's, Steve and Maureen Smith. I had to knock repeatedly before they answered. I was starting to pass out, so I had to let some fresh air in. I was able to open the outside door and get some relief. Steve finally came out and said, "I smell gas."

"I'm glad I finally woke you up."

"So am I; we could have all been dead." He came over, turned the stove off, and asked me where my aide was.

"I don't know," I admitted

"I'll help you into bed if you want me to."

"Yes," I said with relief.

That first year George Armstrong would come

over and help me with my psychology. When we were finished, I told him, "My aide can't find the time to take me shopping for groceries."

"I'll take you."

We walked, with me in my wheelchair. George didn't own a car. We came back with him pushing the grocery cart. I asked him in, but he said, "Not this time; I have to take the cart back." His grandfather had once owned a store and was always having carts stolen.

I was also grateful for George's help in my psychology course which I passed, but just barely. My other classes consisted of Special Language Acquisition, Developmental Psychology, and two family courses treating parent and child relationships.

I was never able to attend the marriage and family course; the professor didn't want to deal with a handicapped person. Perhaps he didn't know how to communicate this information to me or thought I wouldn't need such education anyway. My communication class was very difficult; I didn't have the prerequisites and the professor wasn't accommodating to my limitations.

The second year at Central Michigan wasn't much better in terms of my aide. It started out with Andy getting married and asking my parents to come after me. I went home because he made me leave for the weekend. From Andy I learned that if one hires someone, he must be sure that he knows his job. Andy should have known that he would need a substitute for the weekend when he got married and should have found one.

Andy threatened to quit all during that final year of college. He was still helping me to get up and to my classes.

He didn't have to quit; I fired him. The final straw for me was being forgotten and left in the bathtub from seven in the morning until one o 'clock in the afternoon. I tried to pull myself out by using the bars on the side of the tub, but I didn't have the strength to do this. I screamed and yelled for anyone to come and help while I sat in the tub. I cried, banged my head on the wall and called out many times. After I yelled, I would listen for a minute to see if anyone heard me, and of course they did not. I repeated this procedure over and over. Another way I tried to help myself was to empty the water from the tub when I became cold and filling the tub with warm water. I did this, I don't know how many times because Andy hadn't even left me a towel. I was so angry. I gritted my teeth and said that never again would he do these things to me. I pounded on the outside of the tub with my fist as I would have liked to do to his face. Andy was lucky I was handicapped; I surely would have done him harm, if I could have. I called and called for Andy. He finally walked in dressed in a robe and yelled in an agitated voice, "What do you want?" Once again I was totally humiliated. As soon as he helped me out of the tub and to get dressed, I told him he was fired. He laughed as he left for his apartment.

When I called my social worker, he was totally unsympathetic and had a fit; he thought I should keep Andy. I often wonder what he would have done if he had been in my place. The indignity of not being able to get out to use the toilet was just too much. A fellow can lose his dignity quickly when his bowels release.

At that time I was sharing my apartment with Claude Canter. He was being paid by the Commission for the Blind to prepare my meals and clean the apartment, but I only saw him about fifteen minutes a day. He wasn't much better than Andy. The meals usually consisted of something quick such as the oatmeal mush, raw hamburgers, canned beans, and hot dogs. Claude fixed me raw hamburger. It was so under-cooked that I still wonder why I didn't get sick. He was always in a hurry to go somewhere. Even though I had a lot of hamburger, I didn't want to eat it raw.

Every time I brought up the subject of raw beef, he walked out on me. After firing Andy, I couldn't rely on Claude to help me to classes or with personal needs. Fortunately, my old friend George, like a good samaritan, came to my rescue, and for the final weeks of college helped me. They were the best weeks of the year at CMU; I had a friend helping me, and I knew I could depend on him.

I needed a telephone and ordered one. I was the only one with good enough credit to have one installed. I told my friends and aides that they could use it for local calls. Claude evidently understood this, until the last month of the term. I received the bill and the shock that came with it. He had made more than a hundred fifty dollars worth of long distance calls. I tried to collect the money from him, but his family said that he had moved to California and that they had no way to pay the bill. I never heard from him again. I was glad to be finished with my sophomore year.

Several years later, Andy had the nerve to use me for a job reference. He sent the application to the same person who had recruited me to serve as the consumer advocate on the Community Supported Living Arrangements Board. He had no idea I was even in the area. She called to ask me whether I knew this person, and whether he was the same one I had hired at CMU. I finally had my revenge. It was sweet.

7

TAKING TIME TO TRAVEL

We moved again in 1983. This time, as our family grew up and moved on, the house in Frankenmuth was too large. We moved into the suburbs of Saginaw, on Abbe street to be closer to friends and family. Dave was an electrical engineer, working in Southern Michigan. Chuck had followed in my dad's footsteps, after graduating from Ferris, and was a salesman. Pat had finished at Western Michigan and was a social worker in Bay City. Mom, Dad, and I were still together. Kate had finished school and worked in Saginaw, so she could have her own place. My sister found an apartment in the house that my mother's family had lived in thirty years before. Mom and Dad had been married in that house in front of the fireplace. It was quite a surprise when they went for their first visit; it brought back many memories.

To celebrate our move and Dad's retirement in 1984, we decided to take a trip to Colorado. I heard a voice that said, "Go West, young man; go West." I started with many plans and many things to do, but very few of them ever materialized. The things that I had read about were no longer in existence or were marked only by a sign, such as Fort Madison, built in 1806 in Iowa, and Fort Atkinson in Nebraska. In Iowa we stopped at a farm house turned into a restaurant; here I was able to order my first buffalo burger. It was lean and tasted better than any hamburger I had ever tasted. At least that's what I told my father; after all, I had been talking for months how I was going to order a buffalo burger. We were on our way to Colorado to see the Coors Bike Race. Brother Dave is a bike enthusiast and does some racing. This bike race was a warmup for some of the top cyclists in the world before the Olympics. Dave was eager to see some of the best ones entered and to teach us a little about the sport. We were eager to see everything that Colorado had to offer.

Finally, we were in Colorado and on our way into the mountains, past Denver in our new van. When signs proclaimed that there was a tunnel ahead, I said that I could see the tunnel which of course I couldn't, but I always got a sarcastic remark from someone which made me laugh. Seconds passed; we were in the tunnel, and the van stalled. I can still recall being told how my dad had turned white. "This is no place to play games, Dave," Mother added in a panicked voice. (Dave likes to tease her.) The car kept stalling. I could see how dark it had become, and I was a little anxious also.

"I'm not playing games," Dave said with a worried voice. "This car can't take the altitude. I just hope we can make it out of the tunnel before someone hits us in the rear." He turned his attention back to the road that was in front of him. We finally made it out of the tunnel to our great relief and into a town called Idaho Springs. We were all breathing a bit easier. At the garage, a young kid came and looked at the motor of the van. He looked to be no more than twelve. My parents were worried because he seemed too young to understand the situation, but he recognized the problem immediately. He adjusted the carburetor to the high altitudes and had us on our way in minutes.

After that excitement, we decided to have a picnic down by some waterfalls that were near our hotel. We were able to watch the water as it flowed and fell down the mountains. We found a table and ate pizza beside the roaring water. What had started out to be a likely disaster turned into a great time.

We decided to spend the night in Idaho Springs, an old silver mining town, with many of the original small stores. It looked like the Old West, with towering mountains on all sides. The streets twisted and turned into the hills. I was able to go into some of those small general stores and picture how it must have been to live there in the mining days. We walked back to our motel room which was quaint, which meant it was difficult to maneuver my wheelchair. Sometimes these inconveniences didn't bother me as long as I could get the feeling of the old west.

The following morning, strange sounds woke me up. "Dave, wake up! I hear someone outside. Come on; you have to get up now."

Dave had done most of the mountain driving and was still tired. "Why?" he moaned, but finally got up and looked. "There are girls out there, sweeping the road. I guess I'll go for a ride. I'd like to see if I can climb these hills on my bike." And he was gone.

"Are you ready to go?" Mom and Dad asked when they came for me. We were eager to see why pretty girls were sweeping roads so early in the morning.

"We're sweeping for the Olympian racers,"

they said, "this is part of their route this morning."

I glanced at my mother; my broad smile expressed my pleasure. What good luck! The near disaster with the van again had turned out to be a boon. We had parked on the cyclists' route without even knowing it. Dave returned from his ride just in time for me to yell at him to hurry if he wanted to see the cyclists. It was quite a sight to see as they rode passed our motel room. We were close enough to reach out and touch them. "I'd like to get in the car and follow them," Dave said, and we did. We followed in the van to watch the grueling climb up the mountain. These cyclists must have worked long and hard to prepare for this feat. Great leg strength is needed to accomplish this. It was a thrilling sight for all of us.

We had reservations in Dillon at a beautiful ski resort overlooking the Colorado mountains. This resort was modern and the rooms were large. It was a relief to be able to move and rest there. I was happy we were there in July because I never did do much skiing and the hotel rates were much lower in the summer. We spent a day in Vale, watching the cyclist sprint races. These climbs and sprints were the warmups for the Olympics, which would be held in California the following month. The races wound around the village and we sat on one of the curves to watch the riders as they came toward us. We could see from the looks on their faces that they were exerting all the power that they could rally in this stage of the races even though the terrain was flat.

We drove to Fort Collins from Dillon for our next stop. Dave took another mountain ride on his cycle. He came back and told us about a place that he had passed. It was an old rustic building built along a mountain stream and called the "INDIAN MEADOW LODGE." We thought it would be fun to stay there, but I guess that I would have been uncomfortable in a rustic setting in the mountains. One reason would be that it is very hard to control a wheelchair going downhill, and even more difficult to push one up a mountain. We decided to have dinner at the lodge and ate fresh trout from that very stream. It was delicious. Although I don't eat fish, I took everyone's word for it as I ate my steak. It was a delicious and memorable meal, sitting in the old cabin while watching the stream below us. Dave wanted to take us sightseeing after supper. He turned off the road, down a steep incline to a railing. I stood up to this wooden railing and could hear it creak. It was so old and rotten that if a car hit it, I don't believe it would have kept the car from rolling down the side of the mountain. I didn't sit down even though my parents were insisting I should. There was something inside of me that needed to try to look.

The view was breathtaking, even though I

couldn't see much of the mountains. "Isn't it impressive?" Dave said, as he raised my chin trying to help me see. I thought, "There he goes again, using a fancy word. " We started back the way we had just come and arrived shortly after dark.

I was up early the following morning because I really wanted an authentic cowboy hat. Dave went cycling, and the rest of us went sightseeing. We found Chisolm's, a store in Fort Collins, and I left wearing a suede jacket and my treasured hat.

Cheyenne, Wyoming was our next stop. Alas, we came to Frontier Days a week early. I wanted to see and hear the Busting Bronco Show and the covered wagon race. This show is so famous that we were unable to get accommodations within a hundred miles. But, we were able to see the grounds being readied, such as the riding rings and the Indians setting up their tents. We had a good time and caught the feeling of the show anyway. I was able to buy a "Cheyenne Days" poster signed by the artist and a saddle blanket at the arena.   We took the van up to Leadville, the highest city in the United States, at 10,200 feet. The van was balking again at the altitude. "Turn around, Dave," Mother and Dad kept insisting. I urged Dave to keep on going. As usual, my mother kept reminding Dave to keep his eyes on the road. We finally made it and stopped at an old saloon, to get Dad a beer and calm him down. Miners used to come on their burros into the bar, and there was a picture on the wall to prove it. There were bullet holes in the tables. Dad was still a nervous wreck and wanted to go downhill. He wouldn't even go to the opera house when we suggested it.

"I'm leaving now; you can come with me or walk back," he said. We left with him.

In Colorado we met a couple from Michigan who ran a Jeep tour. I was able to get into the jeep and go with them above the timber line. During the trip they explained the life the mining prospectors led in those early days. Our guides lived in an abandoned miner's cabin, without electricity or water. They carried all their water from a nearby stream. The forest provided the heat for their cabin in cold weather. Their situation made me wonder how the pioneers ever made it through those mountains with their rickety old wagons. They must have been very courageous and determined. When they corresponded with their families back east, a letter may have read as follows:

Dear Uncle Sam,

Just a note to tell you we are all well and hope we are about half way across the country. Soon we will be entering the mountains on our way to California. The trip is long and boring; it is a treat to be able to bathe and change our clothes. Even a hot meal seems a treat. The others in the wagon train are congenial most of the time. We are able to work together to make this passage as safe as possible.

We had a little excitement this gray and cloudy morning. I went out to feed and hook up the live stock so we could continue our trip west. On the horizon, out of the corner of my eye, I saw what looked to be a band of Indians and could hear their drums. I ran to the wagons, yelling, "Indians", and grabbed my rifle to protect my family. I called my wife, Sarah, to bring the ammunition and ordered the children to stay back in the wagon. By the time we were ready to leave, the braves had returned to their tribe and their lodge, or so we hoped. It was a close call, but don't tell Aunt Milly.

It is much more difficult to make this trip than I expected, but we are excited with every mile that passes.

Sarah will write again when we are near enough to an outpost to mail a letter to you. Our best to all of you.

> *Kurt.*

I would have liked to follow in the footsteps of these brave pioneers and taken a trip on one of the wagon trips offered by several companies in the West. They weren't accessible to me and my family wasn't interested in seeing Colorado this way. We returned to our Abbe Street home after two weeks of traveling.

While living on Abbe I had my first chance to join the working force. I called my Aunt Jacquie and Uncle Jack in the fall of 1985 and asked whether I could help in their apple barns. They gave me the job of sorting apples into three different sizes, using a sorting machine. I also helped make cider. I started in the morning and worked late. Dad took me and Mother picked me up. Later, Dennis, my cousin, picked me up.

The apples weren't as sweet or as plentiful as they would be later in the fall. My uncle added some pears to the apples to make the cider sweeter. I asked Aunt Jacquie to pay me in apples. I negotiated with her how many I was to be paid. We came up with a figure of one bushel of number one apples and two gallons of cider. In late fall the barns became cold and damp, but the sorting and making of cider still had to be done, and I was there to help. Mother and Dad helped one day, but it wasn't for them. They didn't accompany me out to my place of work after that. The work was not as hard as they made it out to be. It was my first work experience and I thank Aunt Jacquie for it. We moved shortly after that, so my career at the apple barn was cut short.

Our original plan was never to move from Abbe. Mom and Dad redecorated and even had the kitchen remodeled to their taste. Nevertheless, this wasn't enough to keep us there. We missed the woods and water, the sound of frogs croaking and birds singing. We had always lived in the woods where these sounds were plentiful.

We had sold our chalet in Canadian Lakes in 1983; it had gotten too expensive for my folks to have two homes. We had really enjoyed the area and missed it.

We sat down and discussed moving back to Canadian Lakes permanently, away from the hustle and bustle of the city. We agreed that that was the area we wanted to settle in. So, in 1986, we moved back to Canadian Lakes.

Again we decided to celebrate our move to Mecosta County with another vacation. Any excuse would have done for this trip, because it would be to Las Vegas. I remember on a cold clear November day we high-stepped out to the car to drive to the airport. My parents, Dave and I had started our trip to Las Vegas. We flew out of Kalamazoo to Chicago's O'Hare airport. It was really surprising that such a large air field had such poor handicap access. I had to be carried in a small wheeled chair up two flights of stairs to the plane. Although the porters were nice and polite in Chicago, I felt like a side of beef when they carried me on board. I remember going into the plane thinking, "Thank God, there isn't anyone here who recognized me."

"Next stop, Las Vegas," the pilot announced.

I leaned back in my DC6 seat, closing my eyes and falling asleep for a minute to dream about all the money I was going to win off those slot machines in the casinos. It didn't take me long to wake up to reality; the one-armed bandits were taking our money. They greeted us as we stepped off the plane. We had come prepared for the slot machines with our quarters, nickels, and dollars. Immediately, I started feeding the coins to pull the handles and the bandits were at work, taking my coins.

Dave and Dad went after a rental car, while Mom and I waited at the airport and played the slots. After the machines had taken all of the money we had with us, we went to look for David and Dad. They didn't come for two more hours. We were eager to see the Strip, our hotel, and more slots.

I didn't lose any time getting to my first casino. I didn't need sleep or food. I just wanted to see how much my one-armed bandit could take from me. I named him Jesse, for Jesse James that notorious western bandit. I was equal to everyone. I could pull that lever as fast as anyone else. After a few days, my arms were showing improvement in strength and staying power. The bandits followed me wherever I went. "Here comes dinner," they yelled when they saw me coming.

I did win three cups of silver dollars at the

Silver Nugget. My father kept ordering another free Heinekin beer and urged me to keep on playing. I wanted to win even more, who doesn't, and kept feeding my money in. Of course, I lost all that I had won. I didn't need any encouragement. I was on a mission to rob the one-armed bandits. I went from casino to casino, trying to find just one generous one.

I talked to the machines if I wasn't winning and felt like a bonehead making conversation with the fiends. I wouldn't listen to my brother. He had won ten dollars and quit. He kept prodding me to go to bed, or at least to another casino. I told him that I wasn't tired yet and kept on playing.

We went to Caesar's Palace for a Sunday Brunch. I recommend it. The employees treat handicapped people as though they are Caesar. We all ate until we were too full to move. The food was exceptionally good. We chose from a variety of foods, such as bagels, blintzes, muffins, cinnamon rolls, pancakes, waffles, eggs, potatoes, and a never ending flow of fresh orange juice. We just couldn't empty our glasses before the waiter filled them up again. Every kind of fruit I could think of was served, such as strawberries as big as plums, watermelon, peaches, nectarines, and prunes. They served all the breakfast meats such as sausage, bacon, ham, chicken and even steak and seafood. Champagne was also served. I'm sure there was even more on the table, and it was all perfectly prepared.

We did take one day off from gambling. We met Harriet and Jim, friends of my mother's from her days in Buffalo, at Kathryn's Landing in Arizona. She hadn't seen them for many years, and I didn't know at the time that they would become my friends as well as hers. Michael Dukakis was running that year as the Democratic presidential nominee. I was elated when I discovered that Harriette and I were supporting the same man. My driver and I had gone to the nursing homes in my area to pass out the forms for registering to vote absentee. I left campaign literature in the day room table for those unable to get out. I gave Harriette my last Dukakis pin. I took it off with a flourish and handed it to her. "You'll need this more than I, if Mike is to win. He needs your state, California." I was pleased when she thanked me and pinned it on her lapel. It felt great that Harriette was able to overlook my disabilities and treat me as her friend. This doesn't happen often; most people look at my handicaps first and me second.

I was enjoying traveling the country now that I had been west, so I campaigned furiously for a southern vacation. My parents were getting tired of the cold winters and so I was easily able to convince them to go and spend some time there.

Hugh Shakleford, a teacher who taught history at Arthur Hill, first whetted by appetite for Civil War history. He taught a course called "The Blue and Grey." After visiting the South, I became a Civil War buff and have read everything about it that I could get my hands on, both fictional and historical.

If I had my choice, I would spend the rest of my life in the South. The weather there is more conducive to the life of a person in a wheelchair. Getting around every month of the year is possible. The people of the South seem to have a less frantic life and are more laid back than those in the North. So I was ecstatic when, for a change, we decided to go south in December of 1989. We were supposed to go to Myrtle Beach, but Hurricane Hugo beat us there, and we ended up at Hilton Head. That was the year that John, our rental agent, didn't show up with the keys. After driving for two days, there was no way to get into the townhouse the we had rented. We waited for a good three hours, calling every half-hour, but to no avail. (John had gone to Myrtle Beach to watch his son play in a high school championship game. In the excitement, he had forgotten us.) About that time, the neighbors came over; these people became our good friends. Debbie worked for a hotel and was able to get us a beautiful room until John returned with our keys. Don helped to build a ramp for me. Their two sons,

Stephen and Josh, visited us every day.

Don and Debbie went bowling every week. I was Don's cheerleader while I observed his bowling stroke. I recall when we went over to his house after another disappointing outing for him. He scored only 130 pins, which was very low for him. He wanted to be perfect. "You're the anchor of the team," I said to encourage him.

"Yes, I was the anchor of our team, wasn't I?" he said in his soft, southern way, smiling at me.

The following morning was the beginning of an exciting day. I sat on my Fortress, a three wheel battery operated scooter, which I called "Ben." All hell broke loose because I was going to the ocean on my own, or so I thought. But looking over my shoulder, I saw my parents running after me. "Let him be on his own for once," I could hear them say as they stopped, turned and started back.

I was happy that I was finally to be allowed to go on my own. Ben had a bicycle-type handle with controls on each side. The right side was used to propel me forward, and the left side was for reverse. I took the governor off and went full speed ahead. It was a great ride for a hundred feet or so. Then I felt as if there was something pulling me down, tugging at me. I had sunk into deep sand. "Are you going to help me?" I called back.

"You dug yourself in; you dig yourself out," was their response, but they did come and push me out. As soon as I was free, I took off again, like a race car. I liked that feeling and went down the shoreline like a speed demon. I felt as free as the seagulls overhead. Then, just as forcefully, the ride came to a sudden halt. I was going down close to the ocean at top speed, six miles per hour, when I hit a ditch that the hotel had dug to drain the floods during the hurricanes. Down I went, falling on my right side. I wasn't really hurt; only my pride suffered. Damn, but that made me mad. When my parents came to pick me up, they teased me about the seagull droppings I had fallen into because I couldn't see the ditch. I thought to myself, "What a fool I am." After they had helped me right myself, I did slow down, but not for long.

Every day we went looking for sand dollars (sea urchins) at low tide. That was the only time we were able to find them easily. I kept tipping my Fortress over.

Aunt Jacquie and Uncle Jack joined us on this vacation in January. We were having a great time. One beautiful morning they suggested that we explore Charleston and the open-air market there. I wanted to go and tried to talk my parents into going. I asked my mother whether she could leave her puzzle and come with us. She rose up so fast that she knocked over the table and the pieces went flying all over the living room floor.

I rode with my aunt and uncle in their pickup

truck. In Charleston I wanted to go on a horse and buggy ride. I had to compromise because I couldn't get into the buggy, and even if I could have, there wouldn't have been room for my wheelchair. We went instead on a streetcar. I couldn't have been happier. We were the only ones in the car. The guide explained all the land marks to us, as if we were on a private tour. It turned out to be a very wise choice for us. I learned much about the Civil War on that one special day. When the ride was over, I was helped down from the street car. I turned and waved and said to my dad, "These southern people sure are nice." He was happy that things had turned out so well for us and agreed that southern people sure were hospitable. It was a great day.

My parents wanted to play golf on another day, so Uncle Jack suggested that we fish in the canal that ran through the plantation where he was staying. We started out about noon; we thought that might be the time the fish were biting. He usually came over and picked me up at our place for these fishing expeditions. I drove my Fortress, hopping on it with a lot of hope that we would catch the big one. I never caught anything but seaweed.

On another morning we were awakened by a loud knock on our door. "Who is that?" I wondered. First, my father woke up. He called for me and my mother. "You may as will sit down, Jack and Jacquie," he said to our visitors. By nine in the morning we were on our way to visit Savannah and to eat at a restaurant called Mrs. Wilkes. This was another incredible visit. We all ate so much that everyone would have liked to have had a wheelchair. The restaurant set a grand table. The food was overwhelming. We sat at a large table with people from all over the country. They served southern style cooking on large platters that were shared with everyone. There were two kinds of meat, dressing, and some of the most delicious sweet potatoes I have ever eaten. The food was so good that every time we had company in the South we took them there for dinner.

We went to a fort in Savanna where Bill Sherman rested his troops in the winter of 1865 on his march to the sea. We visited the grave yard where most of the markers had been defaced by Union soldiers when they were occupying the city. Although I was in a wheelchair and couldn't see very well, I could still feel the cannon and almost imagine I could hear it firing.

We took the Savannah River Walk. It is a walk that passed small craft and souvenir shops. I appreciated the walk on the old original bricks; I got the feeling of the Old South there. In one of these shops I found some souvenirs that really interested me. They were pewter sculptures depicting Civil War scenes. One was called J.E.B. Stuart. It portrays the dashing general, with his famous plumed hat and riding cape, at the precise moment he was hit during the wilderness war. Another one interested me: The Rescue, which shows a member of Colonel James Clayton's Alabama cavalry who, when his horse was shot out from under him, broke his leg. His sergeant had seen the fall and tried to grab him as he rode by. It is his only chance for survival as the Union Army was close. These statues were too expensive for me at the time.

We visited Beaufort, South Carolina, a historical town near Hilton Head. I poked around in this quaint little southern town. I found some handmade cloth-mache Civil War soldiers that I thought would be great to own, but I didn't buy. The town had many old shops along the ocean front. We ate at a restaurant where we could look over the ocean from the porch. What a treat it was to dine outside in February!

Later, Aunt Catherine, Uncle Don, and Cousin Jane came to stay with us for a few days at Hilton Head. After thinking many days about those cloth-mache soldiers, I talked my aunt and Jane into going souvenir hunting in Beaufort. I bought the soldiers, three Confederates and two Yankees: a New York Zouave private, a lieutenant in the Alabama infantry; a Texas cavalry sergeant, a private from Georgia; and the Union captain. They are about ten inches tall; every one of them is wearing a colorful uniform which depicts their section of the country. There is abundant detail such as knives, swords, spy glasses, side-arms, and rifles. I was really excited to finally purchase something related to the Civil War.

A few days later was the coldest day I can remember in the South. That was the morning that Dave and I went to Fort Sumpter. My parents were playing golf at the Harbor Town Golf Course. I don't know which of us was more miserable. We all had fun even though the elements were against us.

It was February, and I went onto the island just like the Confederates, on a boat. I was a hundred twenty-five years back in time. I was charging the fort. We could look down in the water and see the sunken boats. If I listened real hard, I might have heard a scream or two from soldiers who had gone down with the boats. We toured the fort, which is five-sided and surrounded by a wall six to eight feet tall. I was amazed at the number of bullet holes in it and wondered how anyone had survived. We were able to visit the barracks and see the crude living conditions. I was unable to get up the stairs to the officers' quarters, which is where they now have a souvenir shop.

I was disappointed, but this is not unusual in

my travels, especially during my visits to historical sites. I can understand that these old buildings represent our historical background and should be kept in as original condition as possible. What I can't understand is why souvenir shops of this type aren't available to all people.

8

RECLAIMING MY LIFE

In 1973, my doctor in Frankenmuth felt that I was overmedicated and told me to try and drop the drug (phenobarbital/dilantin) gradually. He had not prepared me or my family for a breakthrough seizure. Up until that time and when the medication was prescribed, I only had what I called funny feelings. These episodes caused me to feel as though I was floating. I never passed out and was able to carry on a conversation although lights and loud noises bothered me. The spells usually lasted for a minute or two.

On Christmas day of 1973, I was eating my breakfast and remember my leg shaking wildly and going numb and then my arm and face followed before I passed out. My folks were completely unprepared for this seizure. Chuck was home from college and he and my dad were able to lay me on the kitchen floor.

Mom and Dad became very anxious and distressed. Dad hollered, "Call an ambulance; no call the doctor. Call someone," he said with fear in his voice.

Mother ran for the phone and fumbled with the phone book. Chuck grabbed it from her and asked, "Who in the hell do you want me to call?" By that time I was starting to come around and wondering what was the commotion was all about. Mother finally was able to call the doctor, and he said to give the medication to me as had been prescribed. We never questioned the doctors, and maybe we should have, but the thought of another grand mal was just too much to contemplate.

Over the years, there were some indications that this drug combination was too strong, but there was no other drug for seizures at that time. It took many more years before any help came. One of my symptoms, my extremely slow speech, could have resulted from either the accident or over medication. I think that the doctors were impatient with me because of my slow speech, and they did not take the time to treat the real problem, which was the drugs because they chose to take the easy way, blaming the accident. Many people have offered helpful advice. I have been to a rehabilitation center in Grand Rapids, Michigan, The Michigan School for the Blind, a Motor City rehab, and the Philadelphia Institute for the Development of Human Potential. I was treated by many doctors, including the one who prescribed the phenobarbital-dilantin prescription.

Then in June of 1992, my sister Pat, a social worker and therapist, attended a conference on seizures. She concluded that I was losing my balance and becoming lethargic because of overmedication. She called and told me to get to a neurologist as quickly as possible.

Until then, it seemed to me that everyone was saying, "Steve, you're getting weaker and weaker." They said I was harder to handle. For example, it would take two people to help me out of bed in the morning whereas earlier I could do the task with the help of only one person who held the chair for me. I was concerned I would have to move out of my home; I was worried that my parents soon would be unable to help me. My biggest anxiety was that I would lose control of my life. My brothers and sisters also said that I wasn't trying, that I should try harder than I was; but I was doing my damnedest. We purchased a rowing machine, and it was helping me stretch a bit. I thought that the more I used it, the stronger I'd become, and that was somewhat true. But the real reason for my weak condition went unsuspected for all those years.

I had asked the doctors whether there were any improved medications for me to take. I was worried when they told me that I had some damage to my liver. They assured me that as long as I was seizure-free that they didn't think it necessary to change the type of medication. Their message to me was, "I know of no other medication that will help more, and all medications carry some risk of side effects."

I contacted a neurologist after Pat's call. Dr. Awerbuch took time to listen to me and explained the possible consequences of changing medications, such as seizures. He explained the likely possibility of one or more breakthrough seizures. I did have several of these seizures as the medications left my brain. I became extremely nauseated and unable to eat. One time, Dad and I were home alone when I had a grand mal seizure. My dog, Chai Ling, ran back and forth between my father and me, barking, trying to get Dad to follow her. When he finally understood, he came to my bedroom where he found me slumped over my desk. I was sitting in my wheelchair and Dad couldn't get my seat belt off to lay me on the bed. Luckily, it was also the day that the furnace was being repaired. Dad left me to ask the men to please help him. They were able to lift me enough to loosen the seat belt and straighten me out to rest. After months of adjusting, I was able to drop all of the Phenobarbital, and later the Dilantin. (I am now able to manage on a very small dose of Tegretol.)

I went to South Carolina again in the winter of 1993 with my parents and David. We drove to Myrtle Beach with great expectations. I had no idea what was waiting for us. The sun came out and gave us a South Carolina welcome. That was all that would welcome us. I heard an ocean liner whistle off in the distance while getting out of the car. "There's a ship just over the horizon, my father said as he looked towards the ocean and pointed, "Can you see it?"

"No, I can't," I said

My Dad took my chin into his hands and tilted my head up. I looked and looked, but all I could see was miles of blue water and sky.

The entire trip was a disaster for me. I was overmedicated the entire time. I couldn't wake up; I spent most of the vacation in bed.

David rented a plane and invited me to fly with him along the Carolina coast. My adrenalin usually kicks in whenever he asks me if I want to go fly. But, this time I couldn't rouse myself enough to put forth the effort to accompany him, and I felt horrible that I had to choose to stay home.

I came home and called Doctor Awerbuch about

my medication. He said that I was probably overmedicated and lowered the Tegretol. He had me reduce the medication every two weeks, looking for a level I could live with. But I went too far when I eliminated it altogether and had two grand mal seizures in a row. These scared my father, but I was all right; I had been warned that this might happen. Finally, the dosage was increased slightly, and I'm now able to subsist on a extremely low dose with no repercussions after six months of adjustment.

Soon, I was standing by myself for the first time in thirty-three years. This is very important because I don't have to be lifted when I am helped to be dressed or transferred from my bed to my chair. I didn't regain my balance, however, and with my poor eyesight, I am unable to walk unaided. It makes me furious that some professional did not offer these changes a long time ago. I lost many years of my life because of the medication foul up; it slowed my progress in being rehabilitated from the injuries of the accident because the medication sedated me. I felt that I was being rejected by my family and the doctors because I was criticized so often and the doctors found no reason for the slow degeneration of my life style.

I now feel as if I'm on top of the world. I can stand up for three or four minutes. Sometimes I feel like crying, but I don't know whether it is from all those years of inactivity or whether it's just from happiness. Now that I have had time to contemplate, I feel as though I have escaped from hell. It feels heavenly to be able to sit at the computer and write the stories that have been trapped in my mind for so many years.

After that I became stronger every day. I was able to find strength that I had never had before.

After I arrived home, I counted up my resources, and I decided that I was able to afford the J.E.B. Stuart sculpture. My cousin Jane and I made about ten phone calls to Savannah, trying to find the store where I had seen the sculpture. When I called, the owner of the store had no patience for somebody with a speech impairment. She said, "I have somebody else in the store waiting." Then she hung up on me. I hope that customer spent as much money as I was about to. Later, I found them closer to home at Pewter Kingdom in my old home town of Frankenmuth. The owners made it easy for me to start my collection by letting me lay them away and pay a small amount each month. It takes me many months before I see them, but the wait is always worth it.

I've become very interested in the artist, Francis Barnum, and have kept up with his series on the Civil War. I felt very lucky to be able to meet him in Frankenmuth, where he signed my piece for me. Another time, Theresa, the owner of the Pewter Kingdom invited me to a luncheon given for Mr. Barnum. My sister, Pat, drove me the hundred and ten miles to Frankenmuth. Only eight other people were invited to this special event. This suited me just fine. Such a small group enabled me to spend some time talking with this artist. I had the opportunity to talk with him about my Civil War manuscript that I'm currently writing. I asked him where I might be able to obtain information on conditions in the South on the home front. Mr. Barnum gave me a few leads and advised me to try them out. He thought that some of the Southern libraries might be able to send me copies of newspapers printed at that time or have other useful information. I had a great time that afternoon and came away with some new ideas for my book. Mr. Barnum was very congenial and helpful. He encouraged me to keep at my writing and made me feel as though I could. I've become a real fan of his because he is so well versed in the Civil War. It was a honor to lunch with him.

9

MORE OF MY FAVORITE TRIPS

When I was about 9 years old, I was excited when my parents asked if my brothers and I wanted to go to an amusement park near our home in Frankenmuth to try the rides. I wheeled myself to the front door shouting, "Is anyone coming?"

"As soon as I lock up the house," my mother answered.

"We'll be there in a minute," Dad called. It seemed like they would never come, although it was only a minute or two.

We piled into the car, "Are we all ready?" Dad asked as he turned the key in the ignition. We were off to an adventure. Anything that allowed me to move freely caused me to be excited and I knew that I would have as much fun as my brothers that day. I was tired of always sitting on the sidelines or having someone trying to make me feel excited with their words.

Dave chose the airplane ride which was simply toy airplanes attached to a center support which allowed us to feel as though we were flying, if only in a large circle. We steered the planes by a rudder in the front ducking toward the support and then abruptly away from it. Dad and Mom yelled for us to stop, but I couldn't and wouldn't. I had to go faster and faster. I almost tipped the whole ride over. It reminded me of that fateful July afternoon when the horse I was riding was spooked, and my family were hollering, "Slow down and jump off," but the horse went faster and faster. The outcome was better on the airplane ride than the horse ride.

It was the first time I experienced the freedom that flying could bring and it whetted my appetite for more. It wouldn't be until many years later when I would have another chance to fly again. I was almost as happy as Dave when he bought his airplane; I knew he would let me fly with him.

On August 23, 1993, Dave took me up for the fourth time, and he let me handle some of the controls. We had gone over the steps that I would be using while driving to the airport and continued while waiting for the runway to be cleared. Then Dave stuck his head out of the window and stated, "Clear, clear for take off." He taxied towards the runway. When we arrived on runway 45, he told me that I would be flying today. That thrilled me. I leaned forward to reach the throttle and he put the mighty yoke in my right hand. I pushed the throttle in, and he read off the air speed. He started the count at thirty knots. As he directed me, I began to pull back on the yoke at fifty-five knots, and when we reached a count of sixty the plane started to lift off the runway. It is an experience I'll never forget because it gave me power. I was flying! Next, I felt the angle and he said, "You will stall the plane out if you don't level out." I pushed the yoke forward and the plane did level off. It was an intense moment; I didn't know if I could fly the plane without the pilot taking over the controls. I felt my stomach come up into my throat and I was crying with joy. I don't know how many other people can say they have piloted a plane blind. I'm waiting to ask my Dad and Mom when they want me to take them up.

Mike was a pilot on an aircraft carrier. He was the one who first got Dave hooked on flying, taught him, and flew me home sometimes before Dave acquired his license. My brother is a pilot now and earned his license in June of 1991. I was one of the first brave enough to fly with him. It can

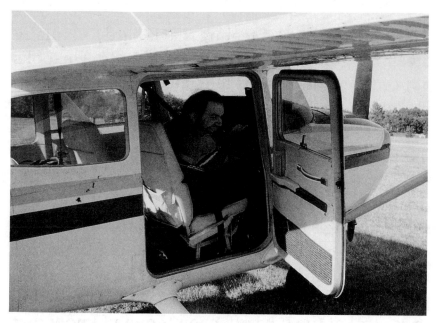

Steve went up with brother David, a pilot, to enjoy a ride over Lake Michigan's shoreline from Canadian Lakes. Steve got to handle the controls during his flight.

be difficult to help someone who is physically challenged into one of those small single engine planes. It is nearly impossible for anyone else, but Dave is determined. I have nothing to hold on to and must be lifted over the wing supports. He grabs me around the hips and with one mighty groan pushes me into the seat. We have a good time, once he catches his breath. He enjoys flying, and I like to come for the ride. I feel the engine roar. He asks me if I'm ready. I know conversation is impossible at this time. I can only nod my head. He is on the radio waiting for an all-clear. It comes and we are off.

Flying gives me a feeling that is hard to explain. I feel free going in and out of the clouds. He looks out of the window and tells me he can see a bird. He lets me help fly the airplane. I take the yoke between my ready hands and pull back on it, and the plane climbs into the ever-changing sky. My brother says to me, "Ease up, ease up on it," and I finally do. The plane levels out like that bird and soars through the crisp blue heavens. That is all one can see out the window and in a small way, one is like that bird. Dave gives me the yoke, and I push the throttle and have the sensation of being in control of the take off, even though I know that Dave only lets me think that I am taking off by myself.

I have ridden with him since October thirteenth of 1991. He practiced touch and go (landings and take-offs) at Grand Rapids and Kalamazoo on that trip. I have been with him as he practices stalls and steep turns. On one trip we followed the Lake Michigan shoreline and then flew east to the small airport in Lakeview near where my sister Kate lives. I let Dave land the plane because I wasn't ready to end my life yet. Flying is fun and exciting.

Our mutual interest in flying led me to push for a trip to Washington to visit the Air and Space Museum. My family and I left for Washington in March of 1992, after calling my senator for some passes to the White House and making an appointment to meet with him in the Senate Russell Building. It was time to make reservations at the Harrington Hotel. This hotel is very old, and we felt as though we had gone back to the Lincoln era. Most of the original architecture was still intact, and the two bedrooms were located on either side of a good size sitting room. The location was great and within easy walking distance which saved my parents loading and unloading my wheelchair in and out of cabs. Most major attractions were wheelchair accessible. Incidently, I never did meet my senator, as he had been called home to Michigan because of family illness. His staff was very helpful and met with us to answer our questions which tempered my disappointment at not meeting with a member of the Senate.

My mother wanted to see our friend, Ruth Lum, and I also wanted to see the historical buildings and grounds. We were very happy to have Ruth as a private tour guide. We visited Arlington Cemetery and witnessed a military funeral. We visited the graves of President John Kennedy, his son Patrick, and brother Robert Kennedy. We saw the Eternal Flame that burns in memory of them. We went to Robert E. Lee's former home which overlooks the cemetery. I was able to see quite a bit of the house on the lower floor. I was satisfied even though it wasn't wheelchair accessible on the upper level. It was very quiet, and I could almost hear him crying out, "I want to return to my house." I could see his ghost walking on his land, or did I see this in my mind? When people are blind, they can see what others only imagine. I could also see Lee sitting in his chair rocking on his front porch. I really don't believe in ghosts, but it did feel as though General Lee was making sure that everything went smoothly. The table, where he ate his meals in the kitchen was set for him. I just knew that he was looking down at me.

We spent a day at the Air and Space Museum. We saw a replica of Lindberg's first plane, named the Kitty Hawk. Dave also took me to see the first passenger plane.

Every time I see a full moon, I wonder what it would be like to walk on it. I would gladly volunteer to be the first handicapped person to fly there. I saw the moon rocks which are kept behind glass. I pictured myself in one of the space suits walking on the moon and gathering these rocks. I finally was able to see one of the first space suits and one of the rockets that powered these early space pioneers into earth orbit. Although I have visited the Kennedy Space Center in Florida, and the space museum in Jackson, Michigan, I enjoyed Washington the most. I became even more interested in our efforts to conquer this frontier.

My spirits were high as I felt the closeness of our astronauts in this museum.

I toured the Early American museum ever so briefly. My mother liked the art museums the most. We needed more time in Washington to explore these two attractions properly.

I visited the Rotunda where so many of great presidents have lain in state. If I was very quiet, I swear I might have been able to hear Mary Todd Lincoln and Jackie Kennedy crying.

Although we had an eight o'clock appointment to tour the White House and were there early, we stood in line for a very long time. We met people from all over our great country, and I had a chance to talk to some of them. Metal detectors blared as soon as I entered the White House. Secret Service immediately pulled me away from all the others, including my family who were told to wait and stand to one side. They covered me with hand held metal detectors. It seems that my wheelchair was the villain. It is reassuring that the White House is always careful and protective of the occupants.

When I finally got into the President's home, I had some good luck. I was taken on an elevator to go to the second floor, and lo and behold, it went down. I put on my reporter's ears and this is what I heard. "The boss is down in the kitchen." I could only guess who I thought they were talking about.

That was the start of my tour. The tourists were divided into small groups before our guide took us through the mansion. First, we went into the formal Blue Room where many of the furnishings were ordered from France by James Monroe. This room was the place where our group was gathered. From there we moved to the Green Room where green watered silk covers the walls of this state room. Great crystal chandeliers hang in every room. Walls are covered with pictures of former presidents and their ladies. We continued on through all the great rooms with the beautiful antiques and pictures. We were very impressed with the State Dining room, but the room I liked best was the East Room. I could picture Lincoln lying in state here. I have heard the President speak from this room, but never dreamed I would be able to visit there.

I thought that my family was going to see Senator Levin. We walked from the Capital building through the underground tunnels to the Russell building. We were able to watch, but not board the shuttles with my wheelchair. The vastness of our government was astounding. We were finally able to find the Senator's office in the huge building. I felt terrible when he didn't show up because it was my idea to see him. Mother made me feel better when she said that dragging them to his office was all right. I happened to be very disappointed because I had come with something for him to read concerning the situation in Russia. I was pleasantly surprised when his aide was very helpful. She was very apologetic that the Senator wasn't there and gave us material about the history of the Senate. We received a copy of the Constitution, directories of the offices of our lawmakers, pictures of the Capital Rotunda and the chambers of the representatives.

I went home determined to take part in the elections of this magnificent country.

On September 23, 1992, I received a phone call from the Clinton/Gore Campaign Headquarters that I wasn't expecting. Charlie, a Clinton aide, asked me whether or not I had yet received my campaign shirt. Sometime earlier, I had ordered a Clinton/Gore campaign shirt that the Democratic Party was selling in order to raise money to fund its presidential campaign. I had written because I hadn't received it. By the time Charlie called, the shirt had arrived. I wore the shirt proudly and I was flattered by the personal attention, especially the phone call. Then I asked whether I could have ten copies of the booklet called "Putting People First," so I could campaign for Bill Clinton and Al Gore. I said that I would like to see Clinton in the White House and to please tell him so. Charlie said he would. I took a deep breath and let it out slowly, then said, "Charlie, if I have a lesser role to play, it's not because of a lack of support for Governor Clinton."

I called the Democratic Party and offered my help using the computer, anyway I could, but I never heard back from them. I am still hoping to hear from the Clinton people.

At the age of twenty, I was so excited about my first vote and voted for the Republican party, which was headed by Richard Nixon. He let me down, and I felt like a fool by his participation in Watergate and by putting himself above the law that the rest of us have to follow. He took my vote and laughed at me and the whole country. I was proud of him only when he resigned.

I certainly was very excited when I heard that my man, Clinton, had won, but not as excited as I should have been. I was numb due and still adjusting to the change in my medications.

Politics interest me and I follow the congress almost daily.

I lobbied in Lansing, the capital of Michigan, all the summer of 1995. This meant going to meetings, sometimes twice a week. The committees were trying to save some of the services for the disabled. The program that I was enrolled in, Community Supported Living Arrangement, had been eliminated in the infamous budget cutting of 1995. We were able to save some, but not all of the services through waivers. I'm grateful for that or my world could have come crumbling down. Transportation is a very big item for persons such as me. Living in a rural area used to make it almost impossible to join the 'real' world, and had kept me quite isolated until I was helped in this area.

In 1994, my family planned another vacation, and this time didn't ask me whether I wanted to accompany them. The truth was I didn't want to travel to the Upper Peninsula because I was more eager to try some new things at home and because I feared that there would be trouble with accommodations

I had convinced myself that I wouldn't have a good time. I went anyway. Mom and my sister, with her three babies, rode in one car, and Dad, Dave and I were in another. While we were riding in the car, I didn't have much to say on the way up there. We were on the road for about six hours, when Dave said, "I see a sign for a casino."

"You're lying," I accused him.

"No! Ask Mom when you see her."

"I will!" I didn't believe my brother. When we saw my mother drive up, it was only a matter of minutes before I was able to ask whether she had seen the casino sign in Christmas, a small town in the U.P. "Dave saw one," I blurted out. "When can we go?"

"I didn't see any casino," she answered. "We'll check it out though, but I can't go today. I have to unpack. Maybe we'll go tomorrow if I can find out where David saw the casino sign."

I was right about the cabins we had rented and wanted to leave when I saw them. I shared a one bedroom cottage with Dave. I wasn't a happy camper. I couldn't get in or out at first until my father talked to Bill, the person who owned the resort. He came right over and built me a ramp, so I was able to enter without someone breaking his back. I still carried a long face with me. The bathroom was hard and nearly impossible because the doorway was so small that my wheelchair couldn't get through and two people had to help me. When my bed in the convertible couch was opened, we found the mattress in three pieces. We tried to hold it together with sheets and blankets. I would have gone back home if it had been up to me. I should have complained,but as usual, I had learned to just grin and bear it. None of the family has suggested that we return, although the resort was located on a beautiful wooded hill overlooking a clean bright blue lake. A wonderful place for other people, but no place for me.

My salvation was the anticipation of visiting a casino in Christmas, Michigan. Mom and I waited all the following day for an opportunity to visit the "one-armed bandits." The rest of the family took the station-wagon to visit the waterfalls. It didn't take much time before my mother said, "Let's take

Kate's car and go without them. We've waited long enough for them to come home." We were off to make our donations to the Indians. Little did I guess at that time that the casino would be the one making the donations. When I was down to my last six quarters my mother begged, "Let's go home now. I'm broke and tired of feeding money into these monsters."

"I feel lucky," I answered, "just one more pull." I put two of my six quarters into the slot machine and leaned back in my chair. I pulled down on the lever. "Win, win," I said as the wheels spun. Bells rang and whistles blew. I yelled for Mom to come. I didn't know what was happening because I didn't know what the flashing lights and ringing bells meant on my machine.

"You've won!" she exclaimed. "You've hit the sevens." I couldn't believe it, but it was true. Finally I was able to smile. My mother was as excited as I was as the casino attendants let the horns blow for a long time. I had all kinds of well wishers. They took my picture. Christmas really did come early for me. I took my money and ran. I had finally won a small jackpot and this was one time that I wished I had put more of my quarters into the slot, but I was happy. It took my mother only a second to remind me that I still owed her for my computer. The trip was a success for me and I smiled all the way home.

10

ACCESS DENIED

To get to the place I am now, writing this book, took many turns of events and fifteen years. Back in the early seventies, I had never felt comfortable with any of my cousins, or my brothers and sisters when they would start talking about high school. I would become frustrated. This was because I hadn't yet entered high school myself. I would sit listening to them talk while tears of anger built up in me. But I tried to never show it. I knew that they had to live their own lives, even though their discussions sometimes left me out. When I finally made it through high school, they were already in college and beginning their professional lives. I was still behind, and it seemed as though I could never catch up.

I had been encouraged to write while in high school and loved it. I felt that I might have a talent for writing. I had tried entering the work force and the normal world through the route that most everyone else takes, but now decided to take a different path. I would use writing to share my experiences.

I first had gone to the Michigan Rehabilitation Center for the Blind in the spring of 1986, but the people there said that computers were not accessible to me. Then in the summer of 1991, Jim Utrip, my counselor from the Commission for the Blind, made an appointment at the Living Learning Resource Center. There, Bob Hill and Donna Heiner, computer instructors for the blind and physically handicapped, provided the first step I had to take to get through the official channels before the Commission for the Blind would pay the $100 an hour that the training at the Rehabilitation Center would cost. I spent about four hours with a couple of nice people who tried and did help me more than they get credit for in these couple of pages. They tested me and said that I was a candidate for Morse code on the computer, but Michigan Rehabilitation for the Blind at Kalamazoo still wouldn't accept me and requested a re-evaluation. Another test was scheduled at the Millet Center in Saginaw in June of 1992, where amazingly, Sue Leonard, an occupational therapist, also said that I was a candidate for Morse code on the computer.

Because I was going to have to run the computer with a keyer, I had to start by learning Morse Code. I made many calls, trying to find a Morse Code Program that I could teach myself. I called the Hadley School for the Blind and requested material. An instructor told me that no Morse program existed at that time. It was then that I called Carol Hubble, a librarian from the Traverse City Library for the Blind. (Carol spends hours researching for me on many topics. She is one person who really makes a difference in my life and has for many years.) Luckily, she had a talking book on the code, and I was able to start before I went to Kalamazoo, where this program is taught to the blind.

On a warm summer night, I started to teach myself Morse Code. I didn't really want to be inside when I could hear my brother and sisters swimming in the lake, but I knew that if I didn't stay indoors and study, I would never have a chance at Kalamazoo. I taught myself by listening to the code on my tape recorder and recording dots and dashes on another recorder. I did this by memorizing the sequence of the dots and dashes for each letter, and then I would repeat them onto the tape. I didn't want to be defeated again, so this was the way I taught myself at our home in Canadian Lakes. I wanted to learn and go forward with some hope. The alphabet took me about three weeks to learn. I had to teach myself a whole new language. It was difficult at first, but now I can send code. A person has to be really dedicated to learn Morse code. For instance, dot-dash is A, dash-dot-dot-dot is B, and dash-dot-dash-dot is C. Once I had memorized the alphabet, I became fluent enough in Morse Code to use it without thinking about it.

Donna Heiner, Director, and Bob Hill, Computer Specialist at the Living Learning Resource Center in Lansing, were the first to take the time to find a way for me to transcribe my thoughts on paper. Donna sent the HandiCODE "Tiny Talk" and "Right Reader" demonstrators, so I could get started learning the computer. And start I did.

Then came the opportunity to learn the computer. I thank my brother Dave for giving me the chance to help myself by setting up this computer with Morse Code and teaching me to use it. He helped me load the demonstration HandiCODE (Morse code program) and Tiny Talk (primitive voice output computer program) onto my 286 system. That was my second step in learning to write this book and many others.

For the first time I had real feedback, even

though Tiny Talk didn't work as well as my Arctic Voice program works for me now. Dave took me and my demonstration HandiCODE programs down to his house. First, he put it onto his computer to help me with Morse Code; he was familiar with the code, having been a ham operator at one time. I can say now that I was very frustrated while learning the computer. At first I had a demonstration program that ran out in sixty minutes. It was disconcerting because it stopped without any warning. My writing would come to an abrupt conclusion.

Jim Utrip, my counselor for the blind, was helpful in getting me enrolled at the Kalamazoo School for the Blind. He has helped to obtain the programs that I need. I did blame Jim at first for not being as quick in getting me enrolled as I would have liked, but now I see, (and that's something for a blind man to say) that he was on my side, fighting for me, trying to help me. It became one of the most frustrating times in my life because I thought that Kalamazoo did not want me back, but I finally realized that I just had to wait for the paperwork to clear. After I saw Bob Hill and Donna Heiner, it seemed that the wheels had stopped turning in the offices of the Commission for the Blind and Michigan Rehabilitation School for the Blind at Kalamazoo. But, they were turning just ever so slowly.

I had a re-entrance date to the MRCB School set for July 1, 1992, for computer training. While waiting, I felt as though they were talking about sometime in the 21st century. Finally, on October 5, 1992, I was permitted to enter. There, a voice synthesizer called "Arctic," and a Morse code keyer which consisted of two paddles, one which emits dots and the other dashes were installed by Bob Tinney, another computer specialist, who is also blind. The "Arctic" translates the code into the written word and reads back what I have written as well as other written materials. As I spent the summer learning Morse code, I was finally able to put words to paper. And I have yet to stop!

While living in Mecosta County, I have had the opportunity and the honor of serving on the Community Supported Living Arrangements Board (CSLA) as the consumer's advocate. I was one of many to be selected to participate in the pilot program. Their support has allowed me to study at Ferris and audit a creative writing course with Dr. Elliott Smith.

My relationship with the Board began when the phone rang, and on the other end was Donna Fraser. "I have called to ask you whether you would be interested in serving on the board of Community Supported Living Arrangements (CSLA). Nothing may come out of it for you, but it would be a help to others if you would serve. We could get more funds to help with transportation and other ways that might enrich your life, if you are interested in the services."

"I will be of any assistance I am able to give" was my answer.

One reason I was interested in the CSLA was to get help with transportation. Bob Curry, my volunteer driver, had quit on me and I was back to depending on my brothers and sisters to take me to the places where I needed to go. Bob didn't understand my slightest needs. Once he took me out to buy a compact disc. When I had the nerve to purchase not one but two of them, he turned on me and started to tell me how I didn't pay him enough, and I should be paying him instead of buying the discs. Mental Health had given Bob a choice of mileage or being paid by the hour. He selected the mileage and then asked me for the hourly pay. He wasn't well, I learned later. His moods would change without any warning. He would be happy one minute and he would become angry the next without any provocation. Once when he took me to Saginaw, in the middle of a thoroughfare, he got angry at the traffic. I told him to calm down and to "Shut Up." His behavior had little relation to what was happening. This kind of behavior frightened me because everytime that I got in the car with him, I didn't know how he was going to act. I know now that his leaving was a blessing in disguise for me. Bob never told me that he was quitting. Once I waited for hours for him to come; but after that I no longer waited...and he never returned.

Now I have made new and lasting friends with people associated with CSLA. Four months after becoming a member of the board, the outreach committee considered me to be one of their consumers. I didn't attend the meeting where I was being voted on. So my name went to the full board minus one, my vote. Next I received a phone call from Sue Poindexter, a board member, and CSLA Coordinator. "I have good news for you," she said. "You have been selected to be one of our consumers." Matt Dussia, another board member from the mental health program, came with Sue to ask me what services I wanted. I selected community participation which allowed me to attend college and my meetings. I have been all over the state attending meetings on health care reform, just one of my duties as the consumer's advocate. I was able to get a spokesman from Representative Dave Camp's office to talk about health care at a board meeting in Mt. Pleasant. Recently, I've been able to have another of our representative come to one of our meetings. Senator Joanne Emmons listened to our concerns. She gave us some encouragement and suggestions to be able to continue the funding. I have contacted our governor and am waiting for an answer or at least a proposed solution to the problems of adult handicapped citizens wishing to enter society.Another of my duties are to help consumers by making suggestions on how they might solve some of their problems by drawing on my own experiences.

The program also gives my parents respite, relieving them from daily chores by hiring a replacement for them so they are able to spend a weekend away from home. CSLA has helped me in buying equipment such as a tub lift that has allowed me to take a bath completely by myself. I'll never again be stuck in the bottom of a tub like I was at Central Michigan University.

In addition, I don't have to feel as though I'm taking advantage of other people to help me because now they can be paid with CSLA funds. Finally, I like the CSLA program is because I'm able to select my own agency, who then sends providers of service for me to interview. I am able to choose who I think will be most compatible with me and able to meet my needs. For once in my life someone else isn't making all the decisions on how I should live and where I can go. I do worry that funds will cease in the government's budget crunch, and I'll have to find another way to live my life.

My drivers, hired through a provider agency,

never missed a day when I had to attend my classes. This was a big relief especially in the winter.

My CSLA coordinators in Mecosta County made sure that I had a driver for my fall term and I had four people whom I could interview for the driver position. I chose two who could take me to Ferris, to meetings and on errands. This is an important part of my life as I live twenty miles from the nearest town, and without a driver I would never be able to encounter others of my generation and would be locked into my parent's era.

As it happens, for a personal reason my first driver had to quit, but I was fortunate to have a back-up who became my primary driver. These people have all been steadfast and good companions for me. They have introduced me to their families, and I can really rely them both as drivers and friends.

I had started my college life wanting to go into the human service field hoping to learn techniques to help others, using my own experiences. I soon found out that wasn't my calling; the world wasn't ready to accept my physical limitations at that level. It surprised me because this was not the case in high school. The local school districts had made allowances for people with limitations and we were usually successful there. But this wasn't evident in the aides I was able to hire, the attitude of the administrations, and the inability to obtain enough people to help me write the papers necessary to secure good grades at the university level in the early 1980's.   This was also before anyone would allow me access to computers. Acceptance of my severe limitations and living and learning conditions at this time were horrendous. · People were so biased it became impossible to continue after several years. I felt that I needed a change in the way I was to go on with my life.

Learning the computer changed my life. This was when I first tried to enter Ferris University in Big Rapids, Michigan. Hallelujah! I was accepted. The world had changed in those ten years and I had found a vocation.

I started Ferris State University on a cold January day in 1994. I had a hard time going to sleep the night before I would begin, but I was ready to go early the following morning. I was waiting for John Bott, my first driver under the CSLA program, to pick me up and take me to my first class. I was getting very nervous. It seemed like he would never come.

I rode to Ferris with him, and I was quiet the entire way. When we arrived, I found out that the school had canceled my class which was another blessing. Because of the cancellation, I was able to get into Dr. Smith's class. I started in an advanced English course that I didn't have the prerequisites for. He let me stay and audit his class. Dr. Smith was another person who took me under his wing and flew with me. I couldn't do the work that was required of the rest of the class, but he helped me to improve my writing skills on work that I had written previously. I had so much to learn and so little time. I attended every workshop he held and was able to receive the one-on-one help that I needed. I also was able to learn a lot from his lectures to the class. If it hadn't been for his understanding of me and my problems, this book would have stayed just a dream. I needed someone like him who wouldn't look at my physical needs and determine I couldn't learn. I had that happen to me at CMU in a marriage and family course. I don't know why the university didn't want me to take it, but I guess the real reasons are that they didn't know how to say "sex" to a blind and handicapped man or that they felt I shouldn't be interested, in my condition. I am glad that Ferris doesn't have those prejudices. Even though Dr. Smith knew I didn't have the prerequisites to take his creative writing class, he accepted me. He was also the one who was able to arrange for my continued education in an independent study program offered by Ferris University.

I started at Ferris in September 1994, and

blithely went in with my stories to Dr. Smith's class. Little did I know how much I did not know. For instance, I didn't know the form for dialogue because I had never seen a script nor did I know how the script should be edited and the placement on paper. I came with everything in paragraph form and in upper-case letters. I've already told you I had never learned to spell correctly, but my computer spell-checker solves that problem for me most of the time. Dr. Smith told me that I only had outlines of my stories and needed more detail. He taught me form and punctuation, which I'm still learning.

He referred me to the writing center and Judith Daday, who has helped to give me a whole new outlook on life. Judith has helped me learn to develop my stories further. I take parts of my manuscript in to her and we work on it together. There are only the two of us; it is a one-on-one situation. She has been able to help me make great strides in my writing skills. Judith has helped me to learn timing and to build my stories with more detail. She teaches about and helps me to correct grammar, spelling and sentence structure. I study for two hours a week. It has proven to be the two most productive hours I have ever spent.

On Sunday, March 23, 1997, I attended an Honor ceremony at Williams Auditorium at Ferris State University. Dr. Susan Hammersmith presented the award to me at the foot of the steps of the stage. At first I didn't think I deserved it, thinking that it was awarded because I was handicapped. I didn't plan to attend. However, Marcia Campbell - Brayton, an academic counselor, explained that it was awarded to students who had earned at least a 3.5 grade point average for twelve consecutive credit hours. I was glad that I attended with my mother, father, and David, who came from Battle Creek, because knowing I'm being honored for my achievements is better than thinking I'm being singled out for my physical disabilities.

I use my keyer to write the text, which I take full credit for, or blame, whichever comes first. My mother does the first editing, correcting spelling, and adding any further punctuation needed. Then I take it to class where Judith critiques it and further helps by explaining the mistakes I made and how to correct them. From there, because I am blind, Mother again corrects the manuscript on the computer. This is one aspect I haven't been able to do; I don't read print. My father has done more than any other person to help me learn to spell. He tunes in his sports on my television and sits by me and answers any questions I have. If he doesn't know the answer, he looks up the answers for me in the dictionary or encyclopedia. I hope soon to conquer these two areas with my new CD ROM. Also my dad is the one who helps me get up early in the morning to prepare for class.

Sometimes it is painstaking work for me, and I spend a minimum of eight hours on the computer every single day. I feel more competent in these areas, but still have much to learn. Sometimes I feel that revision will go on forever and wonder how anyone ever really finishes his or her story. I am more active in the first two revisions, but by the third one I need the ideas of my instructor. She questions me and little by little the story comes out, and I am able to remember more detail. My family has saved many articles about my past, and I bug them until they dig them out so I can refresh my memory. I must make phone calls to other members of my family to get more information. And so my story grows.

Now after more than two years studying under the careful hand of my instructor, I have been invited back into Dr. Smith's class. I feel that it is a honor to be asked. I jumped at the chance to be helped on my books. At first it was hard being criticized on pages I had worked so hard on, but I have become very thick- skinned as I see how much improvement can be made.

Besides my autobiography, I'm working on other manuscripts. To do this research I have extensively used the libraries for the blind in Traverse City and Lansing, Michigan, and also the resources of libraries in New York and Colorado.

This work is tedious and time consuming. Once the cassette tapes arrive, I must listen to a paragraph at a time and then summarize the information and put it into my own words. I am currently researching and writing about Native Americans and the Civil War.

I was very happy when I was encouraged by <u>Accent Magazine</u> to write an article. I sent it in and was surprised and excited when they called to tell me that they had accepted it. I guess that I'm a little impatient because it took almost a year for it to be published. But, finally in January of 1998 an envelope containing the issue arrived. It was the first time that I received a paycheck.

I am all the way back and on my way to being a productive citizen in the community. Finally I feel as though I have caught up to my siblings and friends. It feels good!

11

HEAVEN AND HELL

It can be hell for me to get up in the morning; I never know whether it will be a heaven or a hell day. There have been days when I wonder why I even roll out of bed. Those are the days that I call my hell days. Thanks to my brothers, sisters, parents and friends, there have been lots more heaven than hell days.

My brother, Dave, is only seventeen months older than I am. He has a sense of humor that is wry beyond dry and sometimes sarcastic. In his younger days he liked to make me feel foolish and to play practical jokes.

One time when we were both in scouts, the whole troop was going to go to a local Captain

Muddy television show. At the time I wanted to go, but there was no accessibility for a kid in a wheelchair; Dave went without me the first time. I knew that I was losing a small part of him even then. When asked by the Captain what did he want to be when he grew up, Dave answered that he wanted to become an electrical engineer. It was the first time that the family knew about his goal in life. He was only ten at the time. Today he's an engineer and achieving one of many of his goals. One of the others was to win a bicycle race; he placed second in the state championships in a timed sprint race. Another goal was to learn to fly a plane, which he does. Dave has always been loyal to me. When we were children, he came home every day after school to help with my patterning and my light work. He learned to make slides for the light projector to stimulate the nerves of my eyes. He did this for me even when his friends could be heard playing outside. Dave still comes when I need him. He appears at my door, most of the time within days, after I call him. Dave has joined my parents and me on many vacations and gotten me places that I never could have gone without him. He still comes to take me places that I want or need to go. I know that it is a bit harder for him to get away; he has a family now and lives a hundred miles from me.

David didn't marry until he was forty-three

years old. He married Julie Amundson, who had three daughters from a former marriage: Molly, Johna, and Carly. I was proud that he asked me to be his best man at his wedding. Julie and Dave took their vows over Battle Creek, in a vintage military plane as befitting a pilot. Julie's father, John Amundson, flew the plane for them. I had their wedding gift picked out two years before they had even set the date. I hoped that they would just hurry it up. I gave them a Civil War pewter statue showing a brother carrying a wounded younger sibling in his arms, which I thought depicted the relationship of Dave and me.

Julie's teenage daughter, Carly, had lived with her father, who had few rules to live by. She decided to live with her mother after the wedding. At first everyone was pleased to see the sisters reunited and the family having a stable life. But Carly couldn't accept the routines of the new household or David as a partner heading it. The girls had a difficult time accepting the fact that their mother had remarried. Life became very disruptive for all of them. After a year Carly returned to Nebraska and her family there. She returns several times a year to visit. This arrangement seems to have eased life for the family. The younger girls are adjusting a little at a time. Johna is a very quiet girl and doesn't show her emotions often. Molly is an exuberant eight

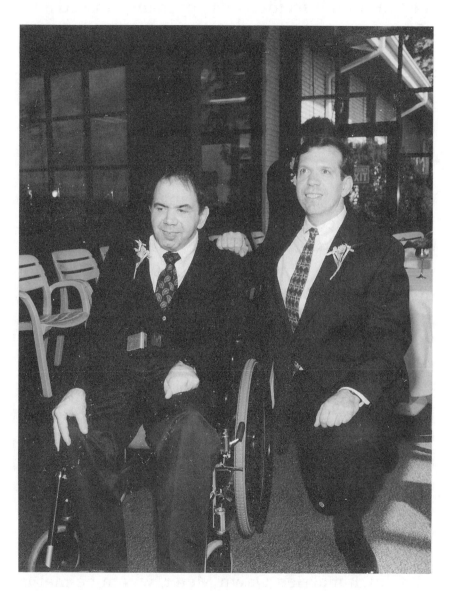

Steve at brother Dave's wedding in 1995.

year-old and has become David's pal.

My younger brother, Chuck, was only four at the time of my accident. He probably missed a lot of experiences because of this. We lived a frantic life in the early sixties, and I doubt that he understood what was happening much of the time. He was still recruited to help, and was often asked attend to the babies while he was still growing up himself. Chuck was never able to accept me in a wheelchair. He always thought I could do more myself. This was very upsetting to me and made me angry because I knew that I was doing all I could for myself. I think he has finally accepted me as I am. Now we go places together. For instance he and his wife, Dawn, took me gambling at the Mt. Pleasant casino at 3:00 in the morning. We played the slot machines until 6:00 A.M. and then went out for breakfast. When he lived in Bay City, he took me to the fireworks on the Fourth of July. I enjoy the balls of fire and the crackling and booming noises they make. Another time we went to a Tina Turner concert at the Castle near Traverse City. We had to stay overnight and shared a motel room. Because of my snoring, he said never again unless I had my own room or a clothes pin for my nose.

Chuck married Dawn Meier, whom he met in Bay City while he was on a sales call for Stapletons. I stood up for him, figuratively speaking, at their wedding. Chuck has a great sense of humor.

After the ceremony we went outside and were surprised to see a waiting bus that was to take the wedding party cruising Bay City. This was the first indication that something out of the ordinary was about to happen. It did when the happy couple passed out ugly red tennis shoes to each of us. The driver looked surprised when he looked at us in those red shoes. He paused for a moment before he snickered, "Where would you people like me to drive you?"

Dawn wanted to go to the A&P super market for drinks and chips. And to the A&P we went. I can just imagine how we all must have looked to the other shoppers. All of the wedding party disembarked, dressed in the formal wear of the wedding and wearing the red, high top, tennis shoes. But we had a great time. The wedding was indeed a happy time.

Although he has a degree in marketing from Ferris and was a salesman for many years, he has recently changed direction and entered the manufacturing business making refrigerator parts.

My two sisters, Kate and Pat, were born after my accident, and brought fresh breath to our lives.

Finally, my parents had daughters, and we had sisters. That caused quite a few changes around the house. Kate has always been spirited and able to make friends easily. She was also a tease and accepted having an older handicapped brother, never knowing me any other way. As evidence of this, she managed to pull my hair every time she walked past me as she grew up. I still blame her for my baldness. Kate is like my dad; they are both strong-willed people. I think this has allowed her to go on with her life of raising three young children alone. My dad and Kate have typical type "A" personalities that have helped me as well as my sister to get through some difficult situations. Kate likes to think that she is in control all the time, but I know she isn't. She waited until she was in her late twenties to marry; she said that she wanted to do it right and only once. The wedding to Jim Earegood took place outside in a gazebo on a sunny May day. It wasn't long before the requests for money started. Jim wanted to open a shoe repair business and persuaded both Dave and my parents to co-sign a loan for him. Jim even came to me with a idea for a key machine. If I would invest $600 dollars in it, he would pay me every time he cut a key. My sister was the only one who ever paid me anything. This was my first business endeavor, and I learned plenty, like never to loan money to a relative. Even though he soft-soaped me by telling me how much money I would make from the key machine, I should have seen the schemer he was.

Even when Gina was a newborn, it seemed as

though I was seeing her more than her dad. The business was finally established, their first child, Gina, was seventeen months old, and Kate was pregnant with another. At that time, Jim packed up and left. He abandoned his young family and the business. We all lost our investments. To this day he has little contact with his family. The girls cannot understand his lack of interest and blame themselves. Our family had no idea of the devastation a situation like this creates. We all cried a great deal, but Kate picked herself up, established a day care center, and is raising her family. They are great kids. She has given them a stable home and great emotional security. She has a young son now and the three kids live close and have become an important part of our family. Their father isn't smart enough to know that he left the best part of himself with us.

This is one reason that I say Pat, although the youngest of us, was the one who looked after and protected Kate, even as children. She has been a source of strength for us all. She has no pretenses and for as long as I can remember, has had the attitude of "This is how I am, take it or leave it," and is very straightforward. She is much like my mother, another peace maker in the family. She is an empathetic and kind lady, with a terrific sense of humor, perfect as a therapist, and a great source of information for me. We spend time together shopping and going to special events. I can always expect a good time when we go.

My parents say that we all complement each other: all different, but making for a well-rounded family. We remain very close even as we have grown older and moved apart. Rounding out this family and again giving it new life is the younger generation, Kate's kids. Gina, Marissa and Tanner, take us back to our own childhoods, and make us laugh, maybe too much. They are just starting school and we remember how it was through them.

Now for the two people who have stood by me through it all. Dad has been the one who has held this family together when most families would have surely broken apart. He was the one at the time of my accident who told the doctors to go to hell. He wouldn't let them try to put me away as a few of my doctors insisted even though it would have been easier for him. He was determined to fight the odds. This is the way he has charged through life. When the family needed money, he went out and earned it; when floors were dirty, he scrubbed them, and when it was time for me to have therapy, he looked for and found the best available. There was no chore too demanding. My Dad managed his work around my needs and was there for every appointment I ever had, and there were many.

I had a team working for me; and my mom was

the other player on my team. She helped me by being strong. Everytime someone had the nerve to say I couldn't do something she would step in and said it could be done. My mother and I have the same temperament. We are both easygoing people, too easy sometimes. I would call us a soft touch with an underlying toughness. People might be able to sell us on any point, but they better be straight about it. I wouldn't get her angry or say anything against her family. This will make her jump all over you. If there's one thing you didn't want to do, it would be to get her wrath up. She has protected me like a mother bear protects her cub. My mother still protects me from people who try to dissuade me from situations I would like to attempt.

Last, but not least, is my dog, Chai Ling, (pronounced Shy Ling) a Chinese Shar Pei. Pat had called and finally convinced me that I wanted this puppy, so I sold my boom-box to pay for her. I named her after the young Chinese girl who was so brave and one of the leaders in the Chinese rebellion in 1989. The revolt took place in Tiananmen Square in Beijing. I thought that Chai, the dog, would be as brave as her namesake, but she is just shy. The one time I had a seizure, Chai nearly went crazy barking at my parents until they came to see what had happened. She is protective and lets us know anytime a stranger comes near.

Chai cannot handle any change at all and will bark if the neighbor so much as changes hats. I have seen much smarter dogs, but none more faithful or gentle.

I hope that I have successfully explained this last part of my book. Every time I fell off my wheelchair, I wondered if there was a God. Then I remembered that he didn't let me die. I know now my purpose for Him is to keep myself alive. I think writing this book is why I should stay alive.

There are people who ask me questions, but don't wait for an answer, even in my own family. Many times people have hung up on me when I was trying to place an order. Even the phone companies have hung up. My solution has been to call them back and ask for a supervisor. This usually works. There's one notable experience that occurred. One day I called several stores carrying speakers to upgrade my stereo system. However, over the phone the clerks refused to take the time to listen to me. My frustration took me to "The Listening Room." Here the owners were very helpful, I was able to talk to someone who took the time to heed my requests. You can bet that was the store that received my business. They even came over to my house to set up the equipment. Just because a person can't speak fluently doesn't mean that salesmen shouldn't pay attention. Disabled people can and do spend money for their needs and wants. I'm glad that the public has become somewhat more tolerant of people of my condition. Now I shop electronically. The telemarketing sales people explain their products, describing exact measurements, colors and uses. It has made it possible for me to pick and choose and know exactly what I'm purchasing. I just have to pick the phone up and place my order and it is delivered to my door. Although shopping with others is always a treat, no one is able to give me this kind of information.

Once I become angry, my speech gets worse. Learning to hold my temper and trying to relax have made my life bearable, although sometimes difficult. I hate it when people jump in and think they are helping me by saying what they think I mean. They are wrong many times, and then I have to go through the process of correcting them. It's a good thing I have a pretty good sense of humor or I would have blown my top by now.

The reason for writing this book is to show others how worthwhile it can be to take the time to communicate with people different from themselves. If they don't take the time, they will never know what is inside the physically challenged person's head, and we have a lot to offer. If others would take the time and really listen, they would be surprised at how much we have to say. Another purpose for writing this book

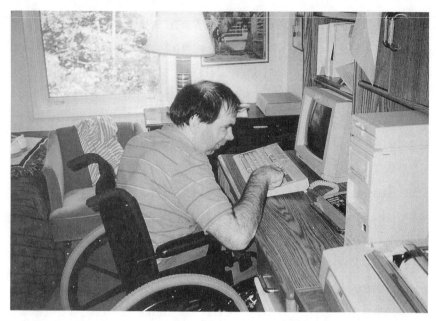

Steve spends up to 10 hours a day working on his computer which is equipped with morse code, Arctic voice screen reader, color scanner and color printer.

is to show people just what I can do with my life. I want them to see that resources are available and there is hope out there. In addition I want the so-called normal person to be open and more considerate to the physically challenged. If everyone would just remember that always being dependent on someone, even to go to the bathroom, is hell, the world would be easier for me and others like me. McDonald's has become a favorite place for me to stop. I'm able to eat my burger and french fries without help, but best of all, they have clean restrooms and are truly handicapped accessible with the doors wide enough and bars in all the right places.

It is hard for the parents of the physically challenged to let them go on their own. I think that if one wants to move out and away from his folks whether or not one is physically challenged, it's all right. I believe a person should be able to have control over his own life so long as he is competent.

Even though I am competent, my accident has so limited me that I haven't been able to go out and find someone who wanted to spend the rest of her life with me. I would love to be married and I feel I would make a good father. Perhaps that's why I love Tanner, Gina, and Marissa, the children of my sister Kate, and Molly, Johna and Carly, the children of Julie and David.

I think that everyone is dealt a certain hand in life. Some are dealt a hand like my own, where it takes a long, long time to find a purpose in life. It took me thirty-three years to find mine.

Although others often look at handicapped people and feel sympathy, they do not realize that they themselves or their loved ones might be in a similar situation one day. I never thought that this could happen to me; even as a child I thought I was invincible. No matter how much care a person takes, however, he cannot be sure that others will take the same precautions; one might always become the victim of negligence. But one should never give up, not even if one has to climb the highest mountain. A person should climb that mountain, no matter how tall or how large it is, if the opportunity presents itself. I'd be a fool to say that I never think about what my life would have been if the accident hadn't happened. It changed my life and the way I live. It changed my family's life forever. For one thing, we are a very close family and try to look out for one another. Another good thing that came out of all this is it has made us aware of others and their troubles and we have learned to empathize with them and to encourage them in their time of need.

Now that I'm in forties, I can look back on my life. I thought that my life had come to an end, but I have realized that is only the beginning.

THE DUDEWICZ SIDE OF MY FAMILY

My Grandfather Leo's family came from the County of Vilna, the town of Pruzhnia in Lithuania in the year of 1898. Leo's father, Peter worked in the coal mines in Lithuania. He went down into the mines day after day. Peter didn't like his job, but he didn't dare tell anyone. Anyone who complained about working for the state took his life into his own hands. They could be executed by a bullet to the head. Peter was lucky because his Uncle George had settled in America and sent for his three nephews. Peter and his two brothers George and Joseph talked secretly about leaving. Even though they worked for the state, they were able to save enough money to buy their passage. Peter took the money, that the three had saved, to the shipping port. He walked in and asked for three tickets. The man behind the desk looked up and asked where he was going. "Are you running away from someone or something?" he asked suspiciously.

Peter looked him squarely in the face and answered. "No, I just would like you to give me my tickets now." He returned home with the tickets and asked his brothers if they were packed and ready to go.

All of their friends came to see the brothers off. They waved frantically from the deck as the ship pulled out. Peter almost fell overboard when someone grabbed him from behind. He turned with fists clenched, but quickly put them down when he saw that it was the captain.

They encountered a hurricane on the trip. "Everyone below," the Captain shouted. They had a very rough ride.

Peter and his brothers were happy to disembark from that ship in Scranton, Pennsylvania. They headed west to their Uncle George in Saginaw, Michigan. At that time many people worked for the railroad, which shipped coal and lumber from that area of Michigan. Peter with his limited knowledge of the English language headed for the railroad and a job. When asked what he could do, he told them that he could work the mines, and that he knew how to work in the railroad yard. He was immediately hired. When asked if he wanted to know what the job paid, he replied that it didn't matter, he just wanted to get to work.

Peter was working late as a signal man on the tracks with a lantern. He could see that the engineer didn't notice his frantic waving. The cars kept coming faster. He shouted for them to stop, but he might as well have been talking to the wind. The cars trapped him between them and he became a "cripple" for the rest of his life. And so the circle turns, I was to be handicapped, as my grandfather, for the remainder of my life.

Peter had married Eva Popielarz. They had seven children at home and now had no income. When Eva died at age thirty-eight the older children were working and helped raise the younger. Peter and Eva's children were Stanley, Walter, Florence, Wanda, Larry, Peter and my Grandfather Leo. He was born in Saginaw in 1905.

After completing high school, he attended Bliss College. He was then able to get a job with General Motors as a time keeper. He rose through the ranks to the position of comptroller. He had to move his family consisting of his wife Irene Munroe, and children Ellen, Guy and Jacquelyn often to many different states. Wherever the General sent him, he would go. At that time it was the only way a person could move up the corporate ladder. He worked many overtime hours during

World War Two.

He met my Grandmother Irene Munroe at a dance in Saginaw. They married in 1927 and my mother, Ellen was born the next year. He died just six days before I was born. Everyone was afraid that I might be born before the funeral was over. He died from complications of high blood pressure. He had been transferred back to Saginaw in 1947.

I find it interesting that my Grandmother Kate was a good friend of my Great Grandmother Eva. In fact Kate was a bridesmaid in Peter and Eva's wedding. And so the circle turns again. Kate's son married Eva's Granddaughter. They were Gene and Ellen, my parents.

My Grandmother Irene was a nurse, wife and mother. She always had to have dinner ready for Leo when he got home from work, and there always had to be dessert. The preparation of the dessert usually fell to my mother as soon as she was able to reach the counter. They returned to Saginaw for all the holidays and a vacation in the summer for the many years they lived in other parts of the country. My Grandfather always spent much time with his father, Peter, and tried to help as much as possible while trying to raise his own family. It was difficult for the young children to understand what had happened to their grandfather. My mother has always tried to help people understand my circumstances because of this.

When I was old enough to miss having a grandfather, I told my Grandma Irene. I loved her for saying she would be both Grandmother and Grandfather to me. She and I were very close, and she tried to play that role. She lived with us about five years after Grandpa Leo died. She always called me her boy.

THE BECKMANNS

Irene Munroe, my maternal grandmother, born June 27, 1908, and died in 1973, was the daughter of Clyde Allen Munroe, born May 13, 1890 and died on October 27, 1908. My grandmother was only four months old then. She and her mother, Hilda Beckmann, lived with Mae Munroe, Clyde's mother, until Hilda was remarried to Guy Bennett in 1916. They had one child, Lucille Bennett.

My Great Grandmother, Hilda Beckmann, was born in 1890 and died in 1975, and the daughter of Minnie Schroeder and Fred Beckmann. Minnie was one of seven children. These were Helen, Bertha, Sophia, John and Fred. She died in or about 1895 leaving five children; Louis, Alvina,

Hilda, Fred and Edwin.   My maternal great great grandparents were born in Germany and came here as children. When Minnie died, Fred retreated to the Upper Peninsula, and became a bootlegger and lumberjack in the town of Baraga.   He remarried, having abandoned his first five children in Saginaw.   His life and family are still known there, and there is a Beckmann walk every year in September in that town.

Meanwhile Hilda's brother, Louis, at the age of twelve took responsibility for his brothers and sisters. Fred May, unrelated, took this family into his home.   Louis went to work at the Goetz Greenhouse to buy the food for the family. Hilda's Aunt Anna helped the family and remained very close to them. Fred Beckmann died in 1934.

I tell this history of my family because it proves I come from hardy resilient stock.   All were survivors and maybe that's why I have survived and been able to forge ahead. I like to think so.

MY GRANDMOTHER-CATHERINE WEIGHMAN

One sunny day with a blue sky overhead, Kate Jozwiak boarded a boat for the new world. She took the last walk ever that morning of 1885 at age five years, that she would ever take in her native country of Poland.

Katy was four or five when she left the town of Posen in Poland. She left with Catherine, her mother, Vincent, her father, Helen a sister, and brothers Tony and Lawrence. They didn't have even a cabin of any sort. The family had quarters in the cargo bay. All she could remember was looking up, and seeing a floor overhead, and hearing the foot steps of the well-to-do passengers. Her family of six was not allowed to come up on the deck where the more respected were housed. They never saw the light of day for the whole journey, and were treated like cattle. All those below were poor immigrants. Vincent, the father, had to work for their passage to the new world.

Kate boarded the steamship. "Where do I go?" she asked the captain.

"You can stay atop until we are ready to leave port, then you'll have to go below." As the ship left port, Kate hung over the rail waving to everyone until they were all out of sight.

Kate walked across the ship with her dress flying in the wind and tears rolling down her little face, and entered the hull of the ship. It would be a rough trip. She missed her friends in her old country. Kate also wondered just what the United States had in store for her.

The days were long, but the nights were even longer. The boat rocked and tipped in the waves. There were terrible storms. She was able to feel them coming for miles. When she did, she ran to her mom and dad. Catherine gave birth on the way over, but the baby died somewhere at sea.

Then one day, after many months of traveling, the family arrived in the United States. They landed in Buffalo. Her father had to immediately find work to feed his large family. Vincent told them that he had decided that they should move west. He had them gather around the table to let the family know his decision. He held Katy on his lap whenever any big decision was to be made. He pointed to a spot on a map. "This is where I am taking you," he said. He chose Michigan because it looked isolated and not as crowded as the eastern seaboard of the United States. Many immigrants were coming from Europe at that time causing work and housing to be scarce.

That is how the Jozwiaks happened to settle in Michigan. Vincent worked as a railroad maintenance man in the Saginaw area. The work was hard, but it was rewarding to see the trains fly past his home.

It was here that another child, Jimmy, joined the family. Jim fought in World War I. He didn't get even a scratch. He came home and went to work for the railroad. It was an unwise decision. He was killed while working.

Years later, Katy married my grandfather, Charles Weighman. My dad, Eugene, was the youngest of their six children. The others were Florence, Lottie, Ted, Margaret and Catherine.

I first remember my Grandma Kate for her cookies. She always had them for us fresh from the oven. I called her my Cookie Grandma.

Grandma Kate always had supper ready for the family whenever they came in. It was always a hot meal too. We never left her house with an empty stomach.

My grandfather Charles Weighman came from a somewhat larger family. He was of German descent. I never knew him. He died in 1925. He also worked for the railroad called Pere Marquette Railroad Company. He walked home for lunch every day from work. One hot summer day he came running home because he wanted to play ball that day. His step was a little higher. Charles walked a little faster as though he knew this was to be his last day on this earth. He ran to the ball field, and hit three home runs. The third one was the last. Charley never made it around the bases. His teammates carried him home.

My dad was playing in the yard. Little Gene ran into the house and called out, "Ma, Ma, they're carrying Pa home. She knew what had happened before they brought her husband in.

Intuition told her that something dire was going to happen that day. Charlie was 46 years old and suffered a fatal heart attack on the ball field. He left a large family that now had to support and care for each other. They struggled to make a living and all went to work as soon as they were able, in order to pay the rent and put food on the table.

Charlie's father's name was Carl. He married two times. Carl's first wife was Sadie. They had four children from this union. They were Mary, Pete, Leonard, and Charles. Sadie died from pneumonia when Charlie was eleven. It was a sad day in the Weighman house that day. Carl married again. He and his wife, Tilly had five children.

My Great Grandfather Carl came over on a ship from Germany as a young lad. His mother took him to the dock, and said only of the children could go. "We want it to be you, my brave son." The boat pulled away from shore. They headed to the new world in an old rickety ship. Carl looked down at his family standing at the dock, and cried. A sympathetic crew member came over to him.

"You'll need to get to work."

"I don't know what I can do, but I will work." He was only nine years old.

"Can you cook?"

"Yes, yes, I can do that," he answered. Carl made the passage without any further mishaps, cooking for the crew and passengers. He came with only one hundred dollars that was his father's life savings. He knew no English. He was one of the brave ones.

Carl landed in the New York, and had to go through physical and mental testing before he was admitted to the United States of America. An uncle was waiting at the dock for him. Most of the Europeans that came over at that time were German. One of the first things he had to do was find a job. That task was nearly impossible when no one could understand him. That did not stop him though. He was alone, and so he had no one to talk to when a decision had to be made.

When he was a little older he started on foot towards Michigan, but ended up in Pennsylvania, where he joined up with other Germans. They were able to start farming. They were all good farmers because they brought new theories on farming. These included crop rotation and fertilizing. They also brought the knowledge and love of music.

Poor economic conditions in Germany forced

many Germans to flee their mother country and head for the United States. Most Germans were way ahead of other ethnic groups in speaking English. They could speak it well before high school even though German was the primary language used in their homes.

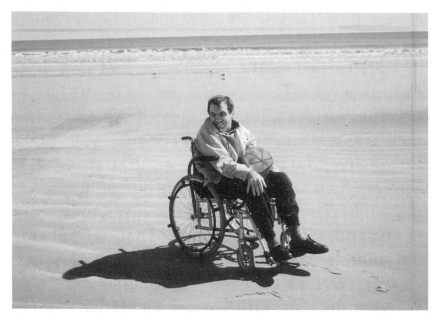

From the front cover, Steve enjoying a day at North Myrtle Beach, South Carolina .

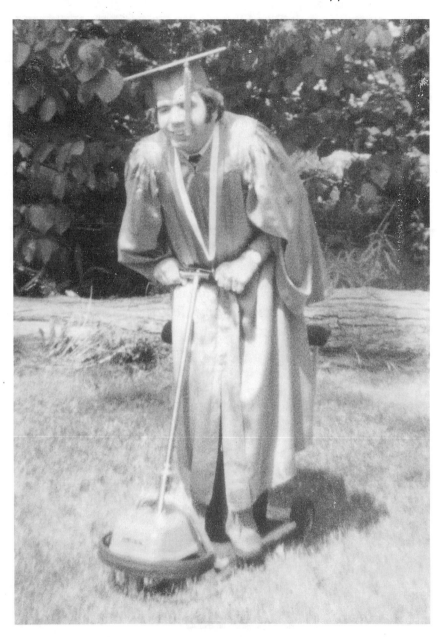

*Also from the front cover, Steve at graduation from Frankenmuth
High School in 1978 riding his Amigo Scooter. "This was one of
my earliest goals achieved," he observed.*

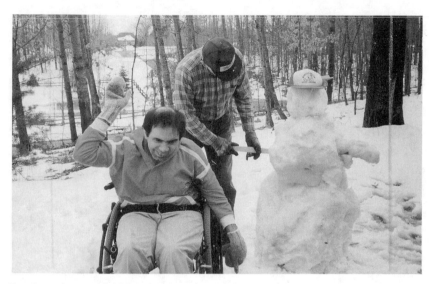

In the winter of 1990-91 Steve and father Gene make a snowman on Easter Sunday waiting for relatives to arrive. Steve had a good time throwing snowballs.

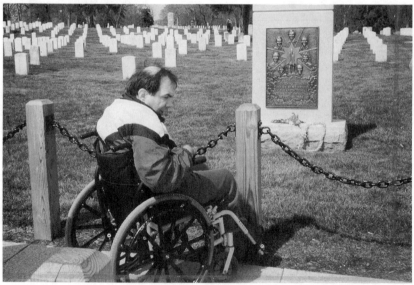

Steve at Arlington National Cemetary visiting John F. Kennedy's grave. John's father, Joe, was being treated for a stroke at the same Institute for Human Potential in Philadelphia where Steve spent five years in and out for treatment.

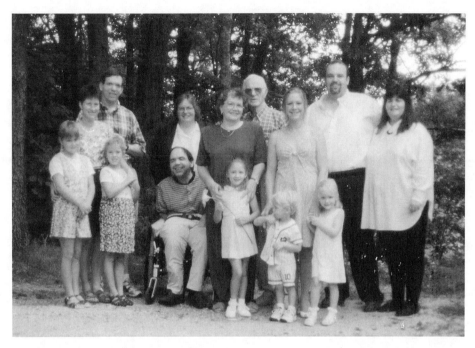

Steve's Helping Hands are his family including brother David, wife Julie and their two children, sister Pat behind him, mother Ellen, father Gene, sister Kate with her children, brother Chuck and his wife, Dawn.

For Additional Copies of

Steven R. Weighman's

Don't Count Me Out

Making the Most of Life With a Serious Head Injury

send check or money order for $14.95, plus $3.50 shipping & handling to:

Blue Spruce Publishing
8442 Small Ave
Stanwood, Michigan 49346
616-972-2234
E-Mail: Weighmans@Centuryinter.net

Michigan residents add 6% sales tax, or $.90 for each book.